I0421370

Workout Guidance

SELECT ARTICLES

by fitness writer Ron MacGregor BSN/RN,

Personal Trainer

DEDICATION

To my companion Magnum

for his

love of exercise

and his

devotion to physical fitness.

CONTENTS

WORKOUT GUIDANCE

FITNESS FOR TODDLERS AND YOUNG CHILDREN, AGE 3 TO 5

CHILDREN'S FITNESS, AGE 6 TO 12

FITNESS FOR TEENS

FITNESS FOR ADULTS, AGE 20 TO 49

FITNESS FOR SENIORS, AGE 50 PLUS

FIT AND SMART

DIET

WELLNESS

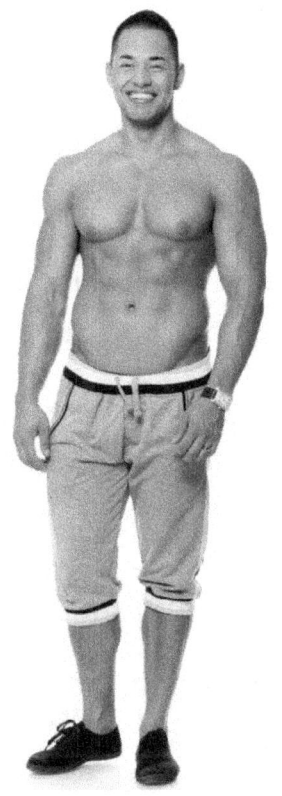

WORKOUT GUIDANCE

The joys of physical fitness

The joys of physical fitness start with the exhilarating feelings that surround your decision to change, plan, and take action. Whether you're brand new to exercise or making adjustments to your current program, you'll be encouraged to know that positive change is always possible.

A few weeks into your new program, you'll become increasingly motivated because you'll begin to see results. Your body's improving physical condition will be enhancing other aspects of your life. You'll notice that every day-to-day exertion is smoother, maybe because your body is processing oxygen more efficiently and effectively.

Moreover, your increased physical strength will allow you to move through your entire world with greater ease. In addition, with improvements in your flexibility, you'll perform the activities of your daily living that require stretching and reaching with less strain.

With a stronger heart and lungs, your brain too will be receiving more highly oxygenated blood and you'll realize that you're thinking more clearly and quickly and your memory has improved.

Maneuvering through life will seem easier and better than ever. Your entire life experience will be more lucid and sensual because by improving the vessel that you have been given for this life (your physical body), you are augmenting its every sense and function, better equipping you for your best life possible.

Now, with all of this to look forward to, you are prepared to enjoy every step of the way. You will even learn to take pleasure in the feeling of physical exertion. With knowledge of physical fitness science and methods, and with a commitment to consistency, you will realize and maintain your own personal joy of physical fitness.

Get ready! Get set! GO!

As you get ready to begin a new exercise program, a little housekeeping is necessary first. If you are brand new to exercise, have a preexisting health condition, are a male aged 45 or older, or a woman aged 55 or older, you should first obtain medical clearance from a licensed medical professional.

Get set! Setting a goal or two will help keep you focused, motivated, and on track. When determining a goal, be sure that it is reasonable, attainable, and measurable. It's important to understand that lofty goals such as losing 30 pounds are best reached through a series of smaller goals. For example, it's better to break down a goal of losing 30 pounds into smaller weekly increments, for example, a goal to lose one pound a week for thirty weeks.

Go! Innumerable studies have shown that the

amount of time you spend exercising is more important than how intensely you exercise, and that amount of time can even be broken into several segments throughout the day. For instance, 10 minutes of exercise three times per day is just as effective as 30 minutes of continuous exercise.

In terms of frequency, exercising four times a week for 30 minutes is more effective than exercising three times per week for 40 minutes.

For many people, starting and sticking to a fitness program with enthusiasm requires a bit more than just hitting the gym. Those seeking to build their fitness foundation and put together a new fitness program can and should first determine what they want to achieve.

You may be motivated to exercise for many different reasons. For example, your physician may have explained to you that physical activity might level out your blood sugar fluctuations, or your motivation can come from simply wanting to look and/or feel better.

Determining what motivates you is a good place to start. Then you can move into a consistent exercise program. Remember that consistency is the key to fitness success.

Before beginning your daily fitness routine, it's important to warm up by doing some mild stretching, deep breathing, or maybe a few yoga poses. Yoga poses can increase blood flow, improve flexibility, and increase body awareness. However, save the bulk of the stretching for the end of the workout. After exercising, your muscles are warmer and can be stretched with greater safety.

Spend five or more minutes stretching, taking special care to focus on the muscles that played the greatest role in that day's session. Try to work up to slow and sustained static stretches (held in place without moving) for 20 to 30 seconds.

Over the course of a week, you should

address three types of exercise to achieve total physical fitness:

1. Cardiovascular exercise for the heart, lungs, and processing of oxygen. Examples include brisk walking and aerobics.

2. Strength conditioning such as Pilates, weight training, or exercise bands.

3. Flexibility training like taking a yoga class, a stretching class, or using a book with diagrams to stretch on your own.

Scientific studies have outlined a best basic fitness foundation, recommending about 20 to 30 minutes of exercise a day almost every day. Again, recent studies have shown that the exercise bouts may be broken into 10-minute segments two to three times a day. Tailoring the type and intensity of activity performed according to your lifestyle and ability is also important. Here are some examples of various exercise types and their associated level of intensity:

- Mild exercise activities include bowling, gardening, walking, yoga, and golf. These are a few of the many pursuits that are especially good for older adults who want to stay active as they age.

- Moderate-level exercises include brisk walking, bicycle riding, and intermediate-level exercise group classes, including moderate-intensity yoga classes. Moderate exercise may be defined as any intensity where it becomes difficult to talk because of your increase in respiration. You can still hold a conversation, but it's difficult. If moderate-level intensity is best for you, and you're the competitive type, then you can join a competitive golf group or a competitive bowling team, or you might want to train for a 5k walk/run to stay motivated.

- High-intensity workouts are for people who have made the decision to increase their fitness level more aggressively. They want to improve their cardiovascular fitness, strength, and flexibility. Most people exercising at the high-intensity level have enough body awareness to distinguish between good and bad pain. A tailored fitness program is usually appropriate here, perhaps enlisting the help of a certified personal trainer, a coach, or other fitness professional.

- The highest intensity training is performed by elite athletes whose intent may be to prepare for a specific sport rather than exercising to improve general fitness. Remember to have fun!

*T*he 48-hour rule of exercise

In a perfect world, we would all get 30 minutes of exercise almost every day. The only problem with this idea, however, is that we do not live in a perfect world! We all have things that we need to get done. We have responsibilities, goals, hobbies, and other plans aside from getting regular exercise. Certain physiological responses to exercise, including the amount and timing of the body's production of important chemicals, lead us to a "48-hour rule of exercise."

So, what should you do if you can't exercise for a perfect 30 minutes per day, every day? A good rule of thumb is to shoot for at least 30 minutes of exercise at least every other day. Exercising at least every other day can maintain and improve the body's metabolism and chemical balance. So, working out every other day will still help you move, although more gradually, toward your fitness goals.

The 48-hour rule of exercise works because some of the metabolic chemicals produced in the body by exercise circulate in your system for about 48 hours before they dissipate completely. So, if you don't go more than two days without exercise, these chemicals will keep your metabolism and body chemistry somewhat elevated and in a more active state. Even if you miss a day of exercise, you don't want to miss more than that one day!

One example of this is that some of these chemicals allow your body to utilize insulin more effectively, thereby keeping blood sugar levels lower and more stable. The 48-hour rule of exercise will help with a steadier flow of energy in your body to better manage conditions like diabetes and even put you in a better and more stable mood.

Some of the natural chemicals released during exercise actually have the same effect in the body as oral medications used to treat type II diabetes. (You should always consult your doctor before making changes to your medication regimen.)

Here is an example of how to structure your everyday workout:

- At the start, it's good to warm up by doing some light stretching of your muscles, which increases blood flow, improves flexibility, and promotes body awareness. Just remember to save the bulk of the stretching for the end of the session.

- Next, perform either your cardiovascular exercise routine or your strength routine, whatever is on your fitness plan for that day. During this routine, the most taxing of the day's workout session is when your body's exercise chemistry is most stimulated.

- It's important that your exercise results in your increased breathing and pulse rate and (it is hoped) breaking a sweat.

The result of this vigorous activity will be a

heightened metabolic rate which will result in burning body fat as fuel for up to 48 hours, whether or not you exercise again.

*M*usic can increase your endurance by 15%

Several studies have proven that exercising while listening to music increases your endurance and improves workouts, like walking, running, bicycling, and other sustained rhythmic activities. In fact some large-scale and important studies show that music can increase your endurance by 15%

Synchronizing your exercise pace with the tempo of the music can heighten your work effort while reducing the sensation of physical exertion.

The subjects of a recent study who cycled to music increased their efficiency and used 7% less oxygen for the same amount of effort that they performed without listening to music. Studies have also shown that runners listening to upbeat coordinated music had an increase in endurance of 15%.

Humans are thought to have been exercising to music 9,000 years ago. Joseph Jordania, an evolutionary musicologist at the University of Melbourne, recently suggested that dancing to rhythmic music was created by the forces of natural selection and evolution.

Moving to chanting and drumming rhythms was a powerful tool that put our human ancestors in an altered state of consciousness (or trance) to better prepare for battle.

Hopefully, you don't think of your workouts as battles, although sometimes it may seem to be a fight to improve your level of fitness. Even in preparation for working out, music can increase your motivation.

Research has shown that listening to music produces a 10% reduction in perceived exertion while exercising at a moderate-intensity level. During exercise, music can make the feeling of muscular effort more enjoyable.

According to Dr. Costas Karageorghis, a researcher at the School of Sport and Education at London's Brunel University, "Music can alter emotional and physiological arousal much like a pharmacological stimulant or sedative." Research has also demonstrated that at the right tempo, music can reduce the sense of difficulty, and boost motivation.

In a recent interview with the *Wall Street Journal*, Dr. Karageorghis said that the sweet spot for workout music is between 125 and 140 beats per minute, and the benefits of music seem most apparent during moderate-intensity exercise. Finding just the right beat is not very difficult because many genres also have music within that range.

The good pain of physical exertion

It's important to learn to distinguish between the good pain of physical exertion and the bad pain that may come from over-exertion or even injury. Critical is paying close attention to how your body reacts to exercise, the amount and type of pain. Observe these feelings both during exercise and in the days afterward.

If you have sore joints, muscle cramps, or the sensation of a strain (sharp burning, sometimes slowly, sometimes all of a sudden) or if you are sore in the muscles for more than a couple of days, you probably have trained too hard.

Not only the intensity of the exercise, but also improper exercise posture and form, especially during strength training, can create the bad type of pain and even injuries. If your goals require that you train at highest intensity, you've got to learn to enjoy the pain by telling yourself that it's necessary for your goals.

However, sometimes the anticipation of pain and pain performing the routine are not worth it for a particular goal. In that case, it may be necessary to adjust your goals so that the level of exertion that you can tolerate matches up to your goal.

The bad pain is what you feel when you might be injuring yourself. This concept should be applied to cardiovascular exercise, strength training, stretching, and any other type of exertion.

Whenever you want to begin a new exercise program, it's wise to consult a licensed medical professional first. People with preexisting health risks, males aged 45 or older, and females aged 55 or older should obtain medical clearance and advice on how intensely it is safe to exercise.

There is always some kind of exercise that a person with any medical condition can perform; just consult a licensed medical professional to find exercises appropriate for your particular circumstance.

You might be motivated to exercise for any number of different reasons. For example, your drive may come from simply wanting to look and feel better, build the perfect body you've always dreamed of, lower your blood pressure, or improve your body's ability to process oxygen effectively.

Determining goals that motivate you is a good place to start; then design an appropriate program that will keep you exercising correctly and consistently. Remember: Consistency is the key to every fitness goal!

Some basic gym terms

Even fitness professionals and experienced exercisers may have misconceptions about exactly what some basic gym terms mean. The following are definitions of words and phrases you're likely to encounter as you work out.

Aerobic/cardiovascular activity:

These are exercises that are strenuous enough to speed up your breathing and heart rate temporarily. Running, cycling, brisk walking, swimming, circuit training with light weights, and dancing fall into this category. The maximum heart rate is based on a person's age. A rough estimate of a person's maximum age-related heart rate can be determined by subtracting the person's age from 220.

Flexibility training or stretching:

> This type of workout enhances the range of motion of joints. Age and inactivity over time tend to cause muscles, tendons, and ligaments to shorten. Be very careful when performing stretches as a part of your warming up are not synonymous. In fact, stretching cold muscles and joints can make them prone to injury.

Strength, weight, or resistance training:

> This type of exercise is aimed at improving the strength and function of muscles. Specific exercises are performed to strengthen each muscle group. Weight lifting and working out with stretchy resistance bands are examples of resistance training activities, as are exercises like pushups in which you work against the weight of your own body.

Set:

> Usually found when discussing strength

training exercises, this term refers to repeating the same exercise a certain number of times. For instance, a weight lifter may do 10 biceps curls, rest for a minute or two, and then perform another set of 10 biceps curls.

Repetition or rep:

This refers to the number of times you perform an exercise during a set, for example, the weight lifter mentioned above performed 10 reps of the bicep curl exercise in each set.

Warm up:

This is the act of preparing your body for the stress of exercise. The body can be warmed up with light-intensity aerobic movements like walking slowly. These movements increase blood flow, which in turn heats up muscles and joints. At the end of your warm-up, it's a good idea to do a little light stretching.

Cool down:

This is the less strenuous exercise you do to cool your body down after the more intense part of your workout. For example, after a walk on a treadmill, you might walk at a reduced speed and decreased incline for several minutes until your breathing and heart rate slow down. Stretching is often part of a cool down.

Tips to help keep you motivated

Sometimes it's a challenge to stick with your regular exercise schedule, and by now you probably understand that the most important key to reaching your fitness goals is consistency. On any given day there are any number of things that may get in your way, and potentially interfere with your exercise plans. It's a good idea to prepare tactics ahead of time. Here are a couple simple tips to help keep you motivated and to help maintain your fitness focus, and achieve the consistency needed for continuing progress.

Sticking with a regular exercise schedule isn't always easy. A common hindrance to your plans is that you just might not want to exercise. You might say, "I'll exercise tomorrow," or "It hurts too much." Keep your fitness goals in mind and know that by working out today, you'll one step closer to better health. Remember when your desire to succeed has been the greatest. This will help you move through your obstacles.

In addition, remind yourself that the key to success is consistency, and it's the times you really don't want to exercise, but you do anyway, that will help build your confidence the most. Try to push through and get the job done. Some say that the hardest part of the workout is getting to the gym, or the park, or the basketball court. With proper self-care, you will keep to your commitment, and, at the very least, you'll get yourself there.

Maybe the obstacle is that you've been working out too strenuously. You may need to reduce your exercise intensity and make sure that you're feeling only the good pain of physical exertion and not any bad pain.

If your goals require that you train with the highest intensity, you've got to learn to enjoy the pain by telling yourself that it's necessary for your goals. However, sometimes the anticipation of pain and the actual pain of performing the routine are not worth it for a particular goal. In that case, it may be necessary to adjust your workout plan so that the level of exertion that you can tolerate matches up to your goal.

Make sure to choose activities that you enjoy and that you will look forward to. Anticipate how great you will feel having reached the longer term-goal. And the pleasure of any day's session, and how working towards it will give you great satisfaction. On any given day, allow yourself to change your workout spontaneously if you're not motivated by the day's workout plan.

Hopefully most of your workouts are goal directed, but even if you don't do your regular routine as planned, any exercise is better than no exercise. It's good to simply get your body moving, your blood pumping, and your muscles stretching as this will all contribute to your overall fitness while supporting your long-term goals.

If you're feeling tired, then have a snack, maybe a banana, some grahams, and a glass of milk, whatever fits your nutritional plan. You can even take a 20-minute cat nap, but no longer because you may find it difficult to get up and get motivated again. This nap option can be kind of dangerous, so use it wisely! Set an alarm and when your nap is over keep your fitness focus and get to your workout right away.

You might say, "I've tried to get fit before and have not been successful." Here you need to realize that eventually you are going to succeed. When you realize your success, you'll look back and remember how you thought you were going to fail, but you made it anyway!

*H*ere's a dumbbells-only workout

All that you really need is a couple of pairs of dumbbells and a bench. A dumbbells-only workout can be great because of its simplicity and effectiveness. The fact is that lifting and balancing free weights, especially dumbbells, increase dexterity and balance.

The ancillary muscles that are neglected when

you are on an exercise machine are more engaged to manage the freedom of movement of the dumbbell in infinite directions. For these reasons, free weights, like dumbbells, can provide more effective exercise than weight machines.

Workout fads and fitness equipment come and go, but as trainers and bodybuilders know, nothing tops a simple set of dumbbells. They are great for convenience, reliability, and versatility when you are trying to build muscle and get in shape.

Beginners should choose a pair of dumbbells that weigh enough to be moderately challenging, but are still easy to control safely. More advanced exercisers will probably want several pairs of dumbbells of differing weights, the heaviest pair being challenging, but easy to manage safely.

Because of the special challenge of balancing the dumbbells, this workout may continue to show you results for many months. When results become less obvious, it's time to raise the dumbbell weight and change out for some new exercises.

Here is a three-day per week dumbbell-only workout that you can do at home or in a gym. Take a one-day rest between workouts. For instance, you could train Monday, Wednesday, and Friday, or Tuesday, Thursday, and Saturday.

Monday

Full body, three sets of 10-12 repetitions for each exercise:

1   Standing dumbbell squat.

2   Dumbbell bench press lying on the floor or a bench.

3   Standing bent-over dumbbell rows.

4   Seated dumbbell arm curls.

5   Standing lateral abductions (lifts to the side).

6   Seated crunches, three sets of 15 to 30 repetitions.

Wednesday

Full body, three sets of 10-12 repetitions for each exercise:

1   Standing dumbbell reverse lunges.

2   Standing stiff-leg dead lift (bend forward then back).

3   Seated dumbbell behind the head triceps press.

4   Standing stiff-leg dumbbell calf raise.

5   Standing dumbbell bent-over rows.

6   Standing dumbbell vertical side bends.

Friday

Full body, three sets of 10-12 repetitions for each exercise:

1   Standing dumbbell step-ups to a stair or bench.

2   Dumbbell, laying on floor chest press.

3   Standing bent-over pull-ups.

4   Standing single-arm curls.

5   Standing single-arm behind-the-head triceps extension.

6   Sitting on the end of a bench or chair, holding one dumbbell between your ankles, leg extensions.

When you can perform 12 repetitions without nearing failure, raise the weight. It's good to rest two to three minutes between each set. You can use this guideline for each exercise. For safety, stop one repetition before you think you are going to fail.

For more of a cardiovascular workout use lighter weights and shorter rests between the sets – 30 to 90 seconds. If you want to perform an additional cardiovascular exercise on the same day, you can do so before or after the dumbbell workout.

Be free from workout confusion once and for all

You'll encounter a myriad of questions and choices along your road to fitness, and making your way can be frustrating and overwhelming. You may wonder when, how, why, where, for how long, and exactly what exercises should I do. With a little patience and planning it *is* possible to be free from workout confusion once and for all.

There is a lot to plan when putting together a smart fitness program. Ask yourself the following questions: How do I start if I'm a total beginner? Or, I'm not a beginner, but should I change my program anyway? Or, Can I just change my current program a bit? Do I need a personal trainer or other professional to help? Will it hurt?

There is a lot to think about, but you can relax, get your head together, and begin by identifying a workout goal or two. Set yourself up for success by carefully identifying a specific goal.

When setting a goal, make certain it is reasonable, measurable, and attainable. Examples include:

- Gain six pounds of muscle in one year.

- Lose six pounds of body fat in six weeks.

- Walk briskly 30 minutes five times a week.

From the above list you may see one that is right for you. These goals do fit our three criteria by being reasonable, measurable, and attainable.

Additional variables that can affect the goal or goals you identify are your gender, age, general health, and experience with exercise, among others. Remember that commitment to exercise and consistency is your key to success.

*O*ust *workout barriers*

When you're committed to improving your fitness, you must avoid any excuses to miss a workout. This can be difficult when someone is trying hard to persuade you to do something other than exercise at your planned exercise time, but don't let them. You'll find that preparing for such a situation will help.

Here are a few tips that may help you oust workout barriers once and for all. Put exercise first on your list of important things to do. Plan where and when you want to exercise. Prepare for any obstacles and then follow through with the workout you planned, want, and need.

Making an appointment with a workout buddy or personal trainer may help with your challenge to ward off possible interference and workout barriers. Soon your friends, family, and co-workers will understand that you're taking care of yourself and are making health and fitness a priority.

An important note on spot-reduction

Although improving the strength or flexibility of a particular muscle group is possible, be aware that doing exercises for a specific body part won't make that specific area less flabby. Spot body fat reduction doesn't work. Abs or hips are commonly targeted as a marketing sales scheme.

Although you may initially lose body fat from your face or waist by chance, the best way to lose is to exercise the entire body without neglecting any area. The truth is, you will tighten up and lose body fat from all over your body at approximately the same rate. Some people tend to lose or gain weight in a particular area of the body, for example, in the face first, while others gain and lose weight from the hips, or from the chest area. Unfortunately you aren't able to choose which area on your body is most effected. Besides it's better for your general fitness to workout your entire body for a balanced wellness.

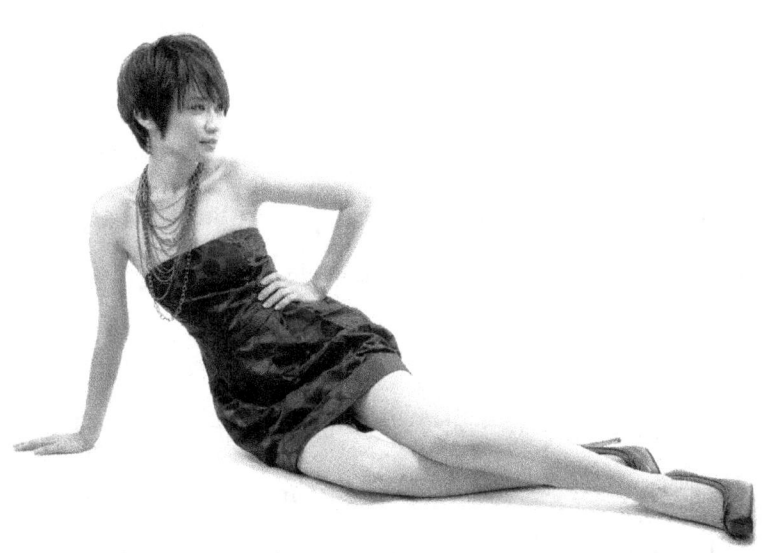

Number-one motivator for weight loss

Whether or not it's admitted, the number one

motivator for weight loss is not better health, but rather it is to look better. An analysis of Internet searches shows that, although exercising and dieting to lose weight is known to benefit one's overall health, it's the idea of looking better that is the under-emphasized motivator to live a fitness lifestyle.

WeightRater.com is a trusted weight-loss diet and fitness product reviewer that studies new fitness trends and compares them to the frequency of certain keywords currently being used in online searches. With the information compiled, it then attempts to identify emerging trends.

In 1997, the World Health Organization (WHO) first recognized obesity as an epidemic. Since then, we have become more aware of the complicated causes of obesity as well as the risk it poses to public health. The obesity epidemic continues mostly unabated and many health professionals report that the epidemic has, in fact, worsened.

Whatever it takes to motivate you to exercise and eat right, whether it's to look better or to be fitter, if the result is that you live even a slightly healthier lifestyle, then that's great!

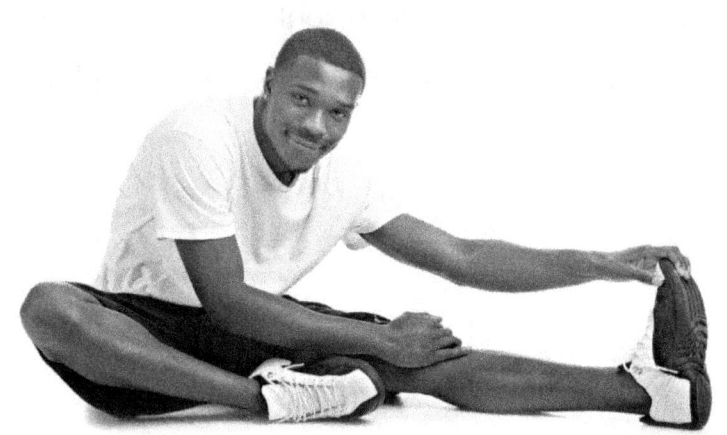

*S*et goals first, then take action

You're excited and eager to get started exercising. You're psyched and wired. You're committed and ready to work out! As you head for the gym, the park, or wherever you exercise, you may be wondering, "What am I doing with all this exercise and why?" Whether you've been training for a long time or are new to exercise, set goals first, then take action. This idea cannot be overemphasized!

Perhaps you could do with some direction. The solution to your problems may be to set a goal or two. Examples of goals you might choose include improving your aerobic capacity, increasing your endurance, greater strength, bigger muscles, and weight loss or weight gain.

When setting a fitness goal, it's best if it satisfies three criteria: Is the goal reasonable, measurable, and attainable? Ok, say you want to lose 30 pounds. Losing 30 pounds seems reasonable, it's measurable, but depending on the time you have to reach the goal it might not be attainable.

Losing 30 pounds is a lofty goal and may be daunting, which is not good for your motivation and may lead to failure. Not being able to see the light at the end of the tunnel makes the goal seem less reachable. You'll find that a better approach is to split one larger goal into a series of smaller goals that are more likely attainable, like "I will lose one pound a week for 30 weeks."

Set workout goals that you know you can gradually and successfully reach. And remember that if your objective is for long-term and permanent improvements, it's the gradual lifestyle changes that will allow you to move into and own these improvements as truly yours.

You're likely to have times of rapid progress and times of slower progress, and maybe even an occasional setback. But, with clearly defined goals, your life-long fitness experience will be that of success.

If you do happen to slip off your fitness trajectory by missing a workout or two, then get right back to it and use any setback as a basis for improvement rather than a sign of failure.

Despite your best intentions, you may miss a couple of workouts or not reach one of your planned goals on schedule. Don't be hard on yourself because everything is actually a step along your path to fitness success.

FITNESS FOR TODDLERS AND YOUNG CHILDREN, AGE 3 TO 5

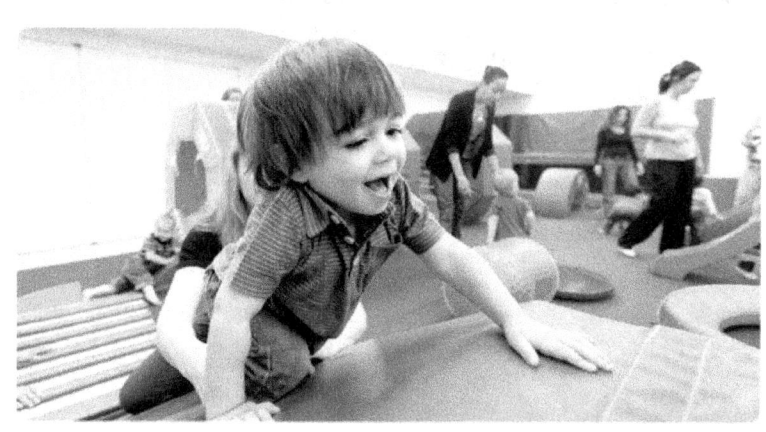

For toddlers and young children, playing generally provides sufficient exercise

Toddlers and young children four years old and younger who can walk on their own should be physically spirited each day for around 180 minutes (three hours), and these activities can be spread throughout the day. Such activities might include:

- Standing from a seated position
- Walking or attempting to walk
- Active games with blocks, balls, and soft toys
- Playing, climbing, carrying, and sliding
- Any type of energetic physical activity if the young child is so inspired

The usual playing generally provides sufficient exercise. And again, praise for the achievement of simple play is solid positive reinforcement for such activity and can be very important in their development. Positive reinforcement may also include a bit of encouragement to simply stand up and be active if the youngster seems sluggish.

Praise is very important for toddlers and young children (age 3-5) to hear because it teaches positive self-esteem. Receiving praise from a parent or caregiver for an attempt to stand, whether failed or successful, can be music to the toddlers and young children's ears. Although most toddlers and young children are active automatically, some need a little positive encouragement.

For life-long health, active toddlers and young children are best served if they are living in households where healthy behaviors, activities, and eating habits are the norm. Toddlers and young children are very observant, and they learn their behaviors from what they see and hear. Just as they develop self-esteem from the praise they receive, toddlers and young children also observe and develop healthy habits based on behaviors around them.

Sometimes the birth of a baby can inspire everyone in the family to live a healthier lifestyle. If you haven't been living as healthily as you want, you may find it easier to make the changes you have wanted for yourself as you bring the baby home. If you decide to do this, it's important to make the changes seem like the norm to the young child. Avoid drastic anxiety-provoking behavior changes like a crash diet.

Make healthier choices gradually and that way the toddlers and young children can grow up in a calm home without the angst of food deprivation or over-exertion, and will experience the good feeling that comes with healthier living.

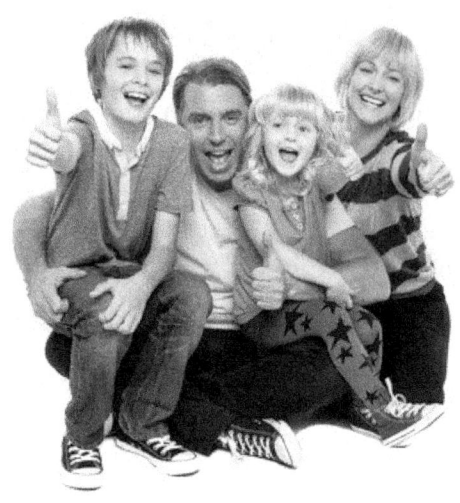

FITNESS FOR CHILDREN, AGE 6 TO 12

The most influential fitness years for children

Childhood is the best time to learn how to eat healthily and be active throughout life. Children (age 6-12) quickly learn by example in what they observe at home and in school. Children are like sponges and they will absorb new behaviors. These are their most influential fitness years as they develop habits they will likely keep for life.

As they learn to choose to be active daily and to

choose healthy foods, those choices become second nature to them. Furthermore, at this age, they can be encouraged to play a little more vigorously than they did earlier in their lives. They may even begin to show interest in a particular activity or sport, or they may not show any interest in a particular activity or sport, and they should know that's OK.

It's important for children to take part in activities that are appropriate to their age, individual abilities, and stage of development. Children should be encouraged to engage in activities that suit their individual choices and aptitudes.

If, for example, after trying out your child doesn't make a certain sports team, it doesn't help to say, "well, next time I'm sure you'll work harder." Instead, say something like "Even though you didn't make the team, I'm really proud of your effort." Sometimes a child's ability level is just not there.

Children should learn to deal with special challenges as a positive rather than a disappointment. This approach allows them to discover what they're good at and what they're not so good at. It's all part of the development process.

Most children need at least an hour of a mixture of mild to vigorous physical activity every day. Regular exercise activity helps children:

- Be calmer in general
- Develop greater self-esteem
- Be better able to focus and learn in school
- Manage a healthy body weight
- Keep bones, muscles, and joints healthy and develop greater strength
- Sleep better at night

We don't want children to sit for too long. These days, children spend more time than ever sitting down to watch TV, surf the Internet, or play electronic games. They spend less time, than previous generations, running, jumping, and playing than their counterparts did 10 years ago.

However, some electronic video games are being designed to get participants up and moving. "Exergames" require active standing, jumping, reaching, and physical challenges through simulation of sports such as tennis, golf, and baseball, among others.

Not only is this a plus, because children are off the sofa, it may even lead to participation in a certain sport in real life. For example, a child who plays active video tennis at home may later decide to join the tennis class at school, or playing a guitar game enthusiastically may someday become a rock star.

Other fitness activities that may suit children include playing ball outside, playing hide and seek, hiking, running, jumping, and learning to swim, just to name a few. If the child becomes involved in a particular sport like track and field, Little League, or kickball, he or she may learn particular exercises to improve performance in a specific sport.

Be cautious when considering competitive sports for children. As young athletes become progressively skilled and competitive, their injury rates increase. Growing bone and cartilage are susceptible to injuries that could hinder or alter development and plague the child for life. Please be careful.

It can't be under-emphasized that for children, it is especially effective to learn by example, as the lessons relate to living a healthier, and a more active lifestyle. Parents can set a good example for children by being active themselves.

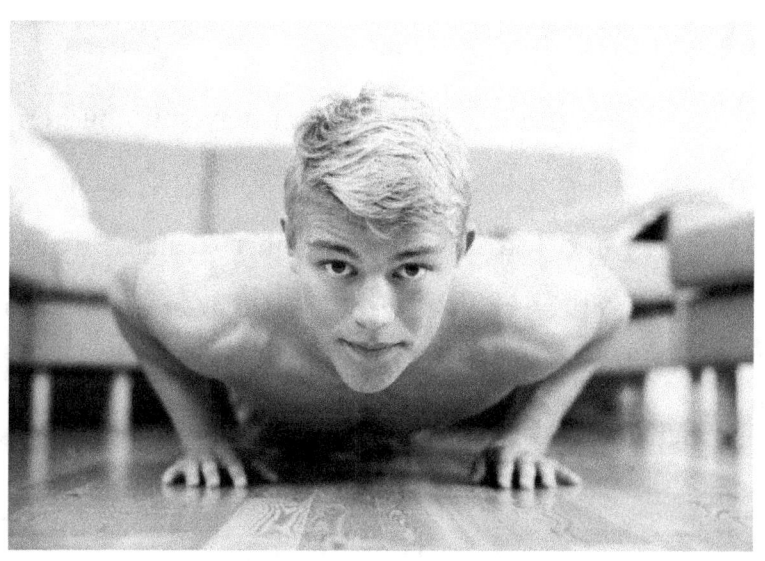

FITNESS FOR TEENS

A solid foundation of fitness for teens

Teens who are preparing for a lifetime of exercise and health, should participate in physical activities that build a well-rounded and solid foundation of fitness. They need a mix of moderate and vigorous activities, for at least 60 minutes a day.

Moderate-intensity activities mean that they are working intensely enough to raise their heart rate and break a sweat. Vigorous activities mean that they are breathing hard and fast, their heart rate has gone up quite a bit, and they are also sweating. Moderate-intensity activities include, but are not limited to, the following:

- Hiking
- Dancing
- Zumba, Jazzercise, aerobics, and many other popular classes
- Brisk walking, jogging, running – whichever is best suited to their ability
- Calisthenics
- Swimming
- Riding a bike fast or on steep hills
- Playing sports

In addition to 60 minutes of general activity daily, exercises to strengthen their muscles and bones, twice a week is recommended. These types of activities put pressure on the muscles and bones that must be resisted with exertion. Examples of muscle and bone strengthening activities suitable for teens include:

- Weight training
- Swimming
- Sports such as gymnastics, football, hockey, badminton, and tennis
- Martial arts
- Calisthenics
- Climbing rope
- Gymnastics
- Power yoga
- Pilates
- Resistance exercises with exercise bands, weight machines, or handheld weights
- Rock climbing

There is usually an overlapping of exercise approach as teens near adulthood, which will depend on the teen's motivation and overall physical ability. It's important to note, however, that teen's bones continue to develop until around the age of 19, and heavy muscle and bone strengthening exercises may not be indicated because of a possible stunt in growth.

Heavy weight lifting, especially if the teen is lifting to muscular failure, can inhibit proper bone growth. Using the teen's own body for strength training is the best bet. Exercises like push-ups, dips, body weight squats, jumps, lunges, gymnastics and many other sports just to name a few are recommended. These exercises are safer than lifting free weights, and are less likely to injure joints and ligaments.

Encourage the teen to wait until past the age of 19 to work out extremely intensely. It will better suit their muscular development and general health.

Good news about teen fitness

If as a teen you're new to exercise, the good news is that you'll progress rapidly for the first six weeks or so. And during this period of rapid growth you may see improvements by exercising for as little as a half hour every other day, and even at only a moderate pace.

For example, taking a brisk walk or using a cardio machine at the gym for 25 to 30 minutes with mild stretching before and after for a total time spent of 30 to 40 minutes is a solid beginning.

As a beginner, you must learn that it's important to exercise at least every 48 hours to better manage blood sugar and other body chemicals that play a part in the body's physical exertion. In other words, don't miss more than one day. Try to exercise every other day.

Once you reach your initial targeted level of fitness, less exercise is required to maintain it. While it's a challenge to continue to raise your level of fitness, maintaining a new higher level of fitness is pretty easy – just get some exercise consistently. Soon as you begin to see results you'll probably want to increase the time and intensity of your workouts.

If you're only able to exercise on Saturdays and Sundays then you should exercise less vigorously than you might want to so that you don't injure yourself. Avoid the weekend warrior injury syndrome, which is caused by not having exercised frequently enough during the week and then jumping into high-intensity activities during the weekend. Just a single workout midweek, including stretching, may help you avoid a weekend warrior injury.

At the beginning, don't stress about exercise and work out too hard, but to see continuing and measurable gains in your fitness levels, after three to nine months, you might increase your workout frequency and intensity.

During the "introduction to fitness period," you can learn more about health and fitness from outside sources like books, the Internet, classes, and personal trainers.

Furthermore, you'll learn about your body by operating it and feeling how it reacts to exercise and different levels of exertion. It's important to learn about the good pain of physical exertion versus the bad pain of physical injury. Learn to notice whether an injury may be developing. It's best to gradually ascend into your quest for greater health and fitness.

🏃🏃

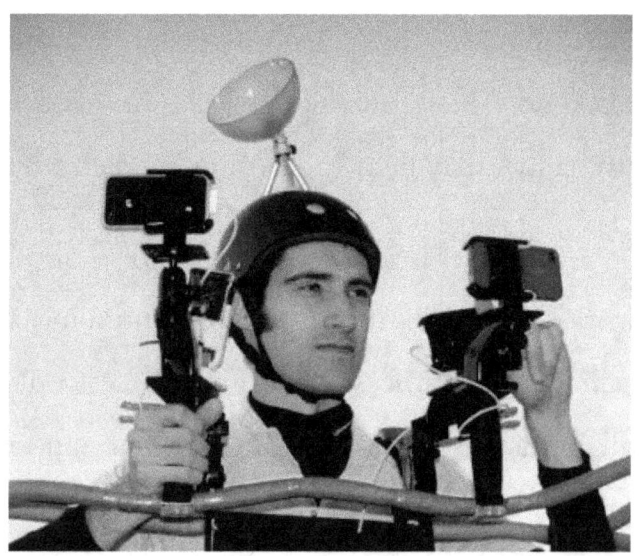

*F*itness gadgets' "must have" features for teens

You can collect oodles of data by wearing a personal

health and fitness monitoring device. Such a device will allow you to observe how your body responds to exercise, your environment, and your body's physiological fluctuations throughout the day and night.

The increase in your body awareness that can be achieved with only one day's use of a monitoring device like this can be very valuable. Wearing it for a few days or even a week can offer you greater understanding of your physiological patterns.

It once took lots and lots of exercise sessions and a close focus to learn as much as you can by wearing one of these personal fitness devices over even a short period of time. They also teach you how to increase the efficiency, effectiveness, and safety of your workouts.

Your personal health and fitness monitoring device will be attached to your wrist, chest, or fingertip. Besides the obvious features like a heart-rate monitor and pedometer, for example, when you shop for one of these amazing devices, make sure it meets the following "must have" criteria:

- It's comfortable to wear 24/7.

- It has a battery that lasts four days or more.

- It gives specific information and tells you what to do.

- It tracks daily and sleep data.

- It can upload data online.

Numerous great fitness devices exist today. Some keep track of what you eat and even your mood. Some can even wake you in the morning at the best time in your sleep cycle.

Some have amazing sensors like an optical scanner to track blood flow and heart rate or a sweat monitor comparing skin temperature and outside-the-body temperature to estimate exercise intensity. Some also monitor calories burned, steps taken, HR, sleep rhythms, and hours slept.

At the very least, having one of these wearable personal fitness devices will make thinking about fitness more interesting. Looking at the data it collects for you may give you motivation to expand on your health and fitness lifestyle.

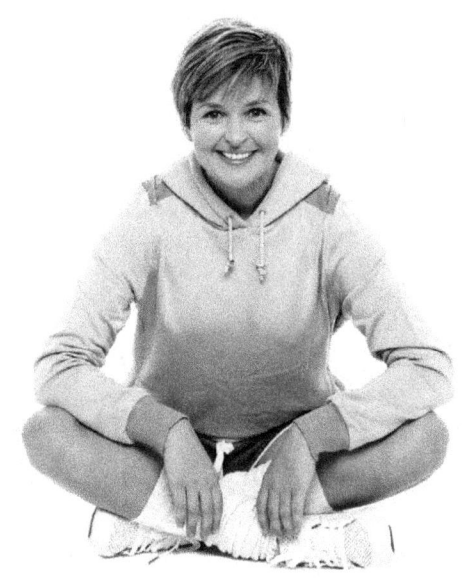

FITNESS FOR ADULTS, AGE 20 49

Adults learn just how much, and how hard, to exercise

Adults are at a time in life when an assessment of just how able, how much, and how intensely, they want to exercise, and to be sure that it is inline with fitness and lifestyle goals. The simple recommendation for already fit adults is to exercise at a *minimum* of almost every day for at least 30 minutes or a total of 150 minutes spread evenly throughout the week. The same amount can be a *maximum* for beginners or those returning to exercise after six or more months away.

The exercise bouts may also be broken into 10-minute segments two to three times a day. Add an additional 30 to 60 minutes of strength training with stretching two or three times a week to make your program ideally complete.

It's important to tailor the type and intensity of exercises according to your lifestyle and ability level. Mild exercise activities include bowling, gardening, walking, beginning yoga, exercise classes, light weight lifting, riding a stationary bicycle, and playing golf.

If mild intensity is best for you, and you're competitive by nature, try a golf group or a bowling team. You might also train for a 5k or 10k walk/run to stay motivated.

Moderate-level exercises include brisk walking, jogging, and bicycle riding (fast or with some hills), medium-level weight lifting, and yoga classes. You'll know you're exercising at the proper intensity if it becomes difficult to talk because of your increased respiration and you break out in a sweat.

High-intensity workouts are recommended for those who have been exercising for nine months to a year and have made the decision to increase their fitness level more aggressively. These people should have gained enough body awareness to appreciate the good pain of physical exertion, while avoiding the bad pain associated with injury.

Specifically tailored programs incorporating aspects of cardiovascular strength and flexibility components will result in a balanced level of fitness.

Individuals exercising at a high level of intensity may want to call on a personal trainer or other fitness professional to help create their exercise program and to coax them past their comfort zones.

Very high intensity and/or professional training are performed by elite athletes whose intent may be to prepare for a specific sport, rather than simply improving overall fitness. However, athletes at any intensity level will make progress more quickly if they enjoy the challenge.

It's best to begin your daily fitness routine with some stretching and a light warm-up to increase blood flow and improve flexibility and body awareness. Save the bulk of your stretching for after the session.

Once you're warmed up, there are three types of exercise you'll want to consider when working out:

1. Cardiovascular activity, such as brisk walking, jogging, bicycling, or aerobics.

2. Strength conditioning, for example, a Pilates class or weight lifting.

3. Flexibility training, like yoga or stretching class. You can also stretch on your own, utilizing books with pictures and instructions.

*A*dult men and testosterone supplementation

Medical experts say that men over the age of 30 can expect to see a reduction in the natural production of testosterone of around 1% yearly. By these calculations, a 55-year-old male could be producing 25% less testosterone than he did at age 30. This decrease in the testosterone hormone can cause a lot of problems that contribute to men feeling differently as they age, and the differences are generally not positive and testosterone supplementation may be considered.

In addition to a diminishing sex drive and lower libido, men can also experience any number of these other common problems:

- Diminishing ability to concentrate, leading to irritability, and depression.
- Decreases in bone density, which can lead to osteoporosis.
- Reduction in strength and endurance, as well as the motivation to exercise.

- Increases in body fat and weight, particularly in the midsection where the buildup of fat can increase the risk for type II diabetes, heart disease, and certain cancers.

- Erectile dysfunction, so even if you get into the mood for sex, which is less likely with low testosterone, your physical parts won't function as well.

Getting older is the most common reason for lower testosterone levels, but some illnesses also can be to blame, including conditions like:

- Type II diabetes

- Liver or kidney disease

- Congestive heart failure

- Pituitary gland problems

If you have low blood levels of testosterone, and you tell the doctor about any symptoms that affect your daily life, he or she will most likely suggest that you begin taking supplemental testosterone. Not everyone with low testosterone will need treatment, but you may want to see a specialist to discuss the risks and benefits if you believe that such a treatment may benefit you.

Supplemental male testosterone may be prescribed and applied to your body as a cream that is usually applied to your shoulders (usually daily), or through injections (usually bimonthly). A less common application, although reported to be very effective, is as a subcutaneous (under the skin) pellet implanted every few months.

FITNESS FOR SENIORS, AGE 50 PLUS

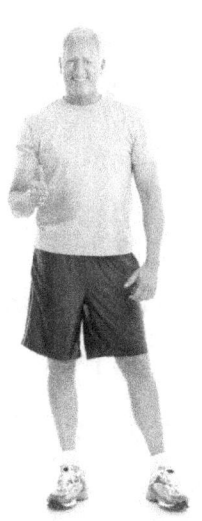

*G*reat news for seniors

The great news for seniors who are out of shape, just a little exercise will make a big difference in your level of fitness and help improve the way you feel. Additionally, if you're already fit, as a senior it's pretty easy to stay fit, or even increase your current level of fitness.

As we age, our approach to exercise will change in several ways. Older adults benefit most from lower intensity exercise. In a fitness program that's meant for senior adults, greater emphasis is put on balance and functional fitness, and your exercise choices will become more closely associated with your medical program and daily activities.

If you're a man aged 45 and older, or a woman aged 55 and older, it's important to meet with a licensed medical professional before you jump into a new exercise plan. Discuss your intentions to exercise and ask for any recommendations specific to your situation and current condition.

Together with a professional, you can plan your safest, most effective, and most efficient program. Whatever your age or condition, there is likely to be some kind of exercise that will benefit you. No handicap, disease, or physical problem will keep you from exercising.

You probably know that exercise can increase your muscle and bone strength and improve your ability to breathe and process oxygen effectively. Exercise can even reduce anxiety and depression, especially if you choose social fitness activities like water aerobics or a walking group.

Essentially, a higher level of fitness can help you remain active and independent longer! When you are ready to approach your fitness level with deliberate intent and action, it is helpful to know the five components to consider when developing a fitness program for seniors:

1. Stamina activities like brisk walking, swimming, or riding a bike improve your staying power, your breathing, and your cardiovascular system.

2. Resistance exercises, like using light weights or rubber workout bands, build muscle tissue, reduce age-related muscle loss, and strengthen bones. Resistance exercise can improve a person's bone density level by as much as 30% over the course of a year.

3. Stretching exercises for the muscles keep the body limber and flexible. This is an opportunity to include a social component to your program, like going to a stretching class. You can also use a book with stretches photographed or drawn, so you can be sure you're doing them correctly.

4. Balance exercises reduce the chances of falling when performing your activities of daily living.

5. Healthy eating supports your exercise habits and overall health.

Depending on your attitude toward exercise and your feelings about exerting yourself, the above five components can be implemented on a sliding scale of effort and ability. Some people enjoy the pain of physical exertion, and some people don't. Which type of person are you? Maybe you are somewhere in the middle of the sliding scale.

If you choose the easier end of the sliding scale, you can simply become more active, while keeping a casual approach. You can also operate with an understanding that it makes good sense to perform activities that use the five components over the course of a week or so. Studies have shown that even gardening increases one's flexibility, strength, and cardiovascular fitness.

If you're on the opposite end of the sliding scale, it's because you're a real go-getter and even enjoy the good pain of physical exertion. You can design your fitness program accordingly. You may write out your weekly exercise plan and keep to it with dedication. You'll probably push your limits more aggressively, and measuring your progress over time may be something you want to do.

Measure your *flexibility* by sitting with legs extended flat and measure how far you can reach. To measure your *stamina* walk or jog a specific route and measure your time improvement. A good way to measure your *strength* progress is that you are able to comfortably do more push-ups (from feet or knees) than previously.

It's important to note that as you age improvements like these must be achieved gradually, over the course of months rather than weeks. Pushing your limits excessively hard and/or too soon will increase the possibility of injury and setbacks. Wherever you are on the intensity scale of working out, exercise *will* produce positive results.

To learn more you can seek the assistance of a personal trainer, wellness coach, or group instructor. It's likely to make your fitness experience more effective and more enjoyable.

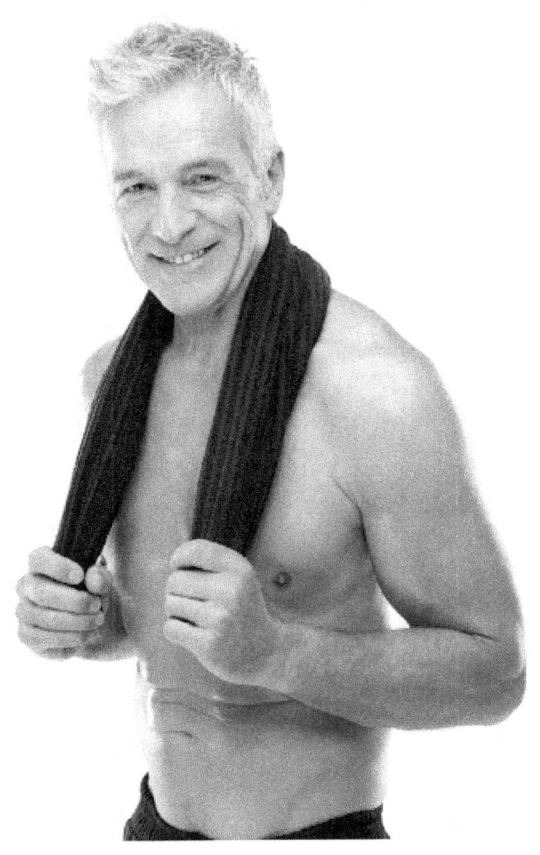

Determine your physical readiness for exercise

If you're a woman age 55 or older, or a man age 45 or older, you should have a checkup and medical consultation prior to beginning a new fitness program, so that you can determine your physical readiness. You should meet with a licensed medical professional to discuss safety factors, possible goals, and any other questions you might have. Plan ahead and before your appointment write down your questions so you don't miss anything that you want to talk about.

Clearance from a licensed medical professional will make your exercise experience more successful. Ask for recommendations specific to your situation and current condition. A professional can help you plan a good program regardless of your current state of health.

Contrary to popular belief, there really are no handicaps, diseases, or physical problems that can keep you from exercising. If after gaining medical clearance you decide that you want some personalized help in getting started, then advice from an exercise or fitness professional like a trainer, coach, nutritionist, or dietitian may be in order.

It is a well-known fact that exercise can help to improve your ability to process oxygen, increase muscle mass, and build bone whatever your age. Exercise can even prevent or delay the onset of adult type II diabetes, cardiovascular diseases, plus, poor endurance, and poor balance. Exercise is good for everyone, and seniors are definitely no exception!

By beginning a new fitness program determine which of the five components of fitness may be of greatest importance to you:

1. Stamina activities, including endurance.
2. Resistance training for basic strength.
3. Stretching and flexibility.
4. Balance to avoid falls and build confidence when moving through special challenges like walking a big dog or hiking.
5. Diet and nutrition, healthier food choices, and food preparation at home and restaurants.

The time you spend exercising and eating healthier is well worth the investment, and you'll find it especially rewarding if you have fun doing it.

Not just delaying the inevitable

Some extremely exciting and conclusive studies have looked at how being fit affects chronic diseases and length of life. "We've determined that being fit is not just delaying the inevitable, but it is actually lowering the onset of chronic disease in the final years of life," says Dr. Jarett Berry, assistant professor of internal medicine and author of the study (online in the *Archives of Internal Medicine*).

This positive effect continues until the end of life, with fitter individuals living their final five years with fewer chronic diseases. The effects were the same in both men and women. These data suggest that cardiovascular exercise such as brisk walking, jogging, or running adds years to your life and also increases the quality of those years.

Fitness is said to compress the incidence of chronic illness into a smaller amount of time at the end of life, Dr. Berry says. This doesn't happen in every single case, but it's a pretty safe bet that the person who is fit will live longer and have a higher quality of life than the person who is not.

Spend 120 seconds to improve your driving

Driving isn't as laid back and easy as we may think, especially as we age and realize that our flexibility, vision, and reflexes are changing. You may be accustomed to driving on a regular basis, so it seems easy. However, in actuality driving requires good muscle strength and reaction time, proper arm and leg flexibility, and general dexterity.

You will find that spending only about 120 seconds doing a few specific stretches before climbing into the driver's will keep you safer. In addition, it will make your overall driving experience more enjoyable.

Hopefully, you've always looked over your shoulder before making a turn or changing lanes. As you were likely taught in school back when we all had driver's education, the combined mirror check and then over-the-shoulder look is safest. I'll never forget those awful driver's education movies that we saw in school, the memories have stayed in my mind over many years, which is probably a good thing!

So, before you get behind the wheel, take just two minutes to do these simple stretches:

1) Keep your legs straight and bend over while putting your hands on your knees for support and then hold the position for 20 seconds. If you can reach lower or can even touch your toes, then do it.

2) With your hands on your knees, lower to a sitting position (upper legs no deeper than parallel to the ground) and hold the position for 10 – 20 seconds.

3) Stand up tall and clasp your hands behind your waist or as close as you can – you will eventually be able to clasp your hands if you can't today – and hold the position for 10 – 20 seconds.

4) Last, stretch the neck. Look straight ahead, then very lightly twist your neck to look over one of your shoulders and then place your hand on that side on your chin and increase the twist slightly and lightly and hold the position for 5 – 10 seconds and then do the same on the other side twisting your head slowly and carefully.

Excellent! Your driving will now be more comfortable and safer, and you will have spent only a few seconds of your day preparing for it. If you feel you need to do the stretches for longer or to repeat them once you've finished, then by all means do so. Performing movements like these before each driving experience will help to prolong your time on the road.

🏃🏃

Bigger and better bones

It happens to all of us. As we age, our bones tend to become less dense and more brittle. As years go by, our muscles, ligaments, and joints become weaker with reduced flexibility. Seniors are the ones who are the most susceptible to conditions like osteoporosis, arthritis, and other bone and joint ailments, but one can take measures to curb these conditions.

This is where exercise comes in. Weight-bearing or resistance exercises will build you bigger and better bones.

Other factors that may contribute to weaker bones include a poor diet, smoking, and what could perhaps prove to be the most dangerous habit of all — a lack of physical activity. It is never too late in life to take up exercise.

Contrary to what one may first think, exercise won't increase the chance of bone injury. It will actually make your bones stronger and also help to improve your overall strength, flexibility, and balance.

Remember, it's always smart to consult a licensed medical professional before beginning a new exercise program, especially if you're a man 45 years old, or a woman age 55, or are brand new to exercise.

Exercising to build up bone density can be as easy as 20 minutes per day doing some simple exercises. At the onset of your new exercise program, you should take into account the areas that can be addressed:

- Current bone density
- Muscle strength
- Range of motion in joints
- Balance

- General fitness

Here are a few of the most common weight-bearing exercises that have proven to strengthen bones and increase bone density over time:

- Walking with light weights, 2-3 pounds is all you need.

- Climbing stairs (climb up, not down - because it's more dangerous and not that beneficial).

- Stair-stepper machines (can be very difficult, but some people love them).

- Elliptical rider machines, rowing machines, keep it fairly light to avoid straining your back.

- Low-impact exercise classes.

Determine what bone strengthening activity you enjoy enough to want to do it consistently.

As part of your pre-workout medical evaluation, consider having a bone density measurement test. Then after working out for 6 or 12 months return for a follow-up test so you can see what kind of progress you've made.

You may be impressed by the results! Some people have shown as much as a 30% increase in bone density after just six months of beginning a simple weight resistance program.

$$\frac{1}{\gamma}$$

Q*uality and quantity of life*

Americans are now living longer than they ever have before. Average life expectancy is 78 years, up from 74 years in 1980. However, are we living better? As you might suspect, eating right and exercising regularly does have as much to do with quality of life, as it does with quantity of life.

The incidence of many chronic diseases, like type II diabetes and heart disease, has been increasing. Although we are spending more years living, we are also spending more years having to deal with chronic illness. Numerous studies have shown that even if you haven't previously bothered with exercise, getting even a little exercise can improve your quality of life, at any age.

To put it simply, exercise and fitness don't just add years to our lives, according to numerous studies, a fitness lifestyle can also help to postpone, or eliminate, the onset of chronic illness.

A longer life was not the only benefit shared by those who exercised more, but the seniors who were the most active also experienced fewer diseases and illnesses than those who were sedentary.

The active seniors who did develop chronic diseases, did so later in life. The most aerobically fit people tended to live with chronic illnesses in only the final five years of their lives while the least fit lived with those illnesses in the final 10, 15, or even 20 years.

Dr. Jarrett Berry, an assistant professor of internal medicine at U.T. Southwestern, says, "Studies suggest that someone in midlife who moves from the least fit to the second to the least fit category will get more benefit, in terms of postponing possible late-life chronic diseases, than someone who moves to the highest fitness grouping from the second highest."

Moving out of that least fit category requires, he says,

"only a small dose of exercise," like 20 or 30 minutes of walking on most days during the week. "You don't have to become an athlete," says Dr. Willis, who himself has little time for exercise, but tries to fit in a daily walk. "Just getting up off of the couch is the key."

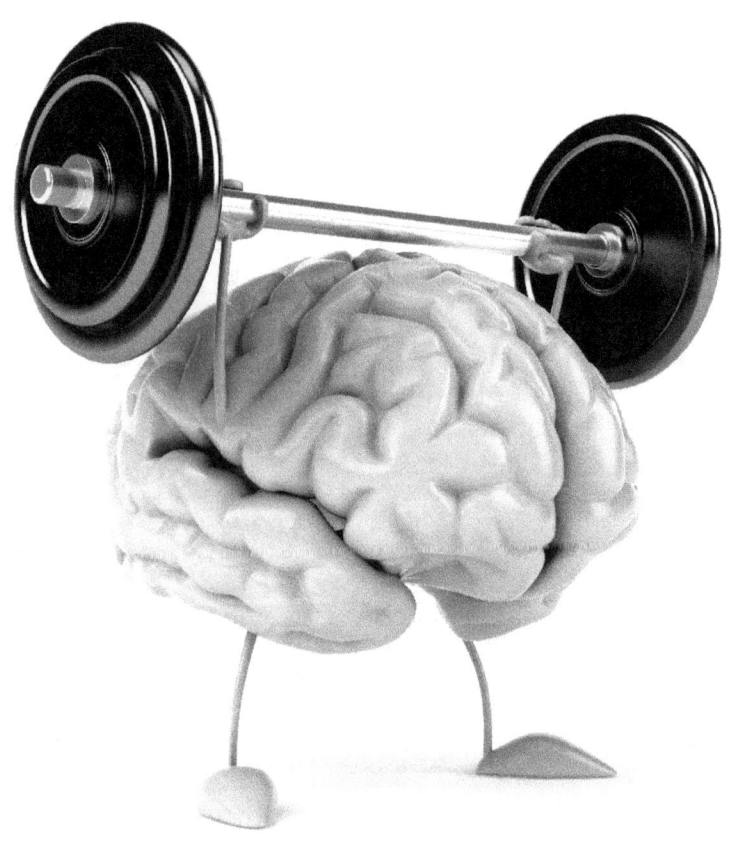

FIT AND SMART

*R*obust brain health

Studies have shown that exercise can greatly improve cognition, especially memory. And for the most robust brain health, it's best to incorporate both aerobic and strength building exercise into your health and fitness program.

Scientists at the Salk Institute for Biological Studies in La Jolla, California, were the first to conclude definitively that exercise actually increases the size of the brain. In these studies, the scientists observed that mice that used their running wheels produced many more brain cells in an area within the brain where memory functions, than sedentary mice.

According to a human study published in the *Journal of Aging Research*, scientists at the University of British Columbia looked at women who had mild cognitive impairment. This means their memory and thinking were less sharp than what would be considered normal for their age group. The study shows that aerobic and strength training improved cognition.

Aerobic training and strength training affect the brain in slightly different ways. According to Teresa Liu-Ambrose, an associate professor in the Brain Research Center at the University of British Columbia, the difference between these two types of exercise is that they target separate areas of cognition. They promote the release of different kinds of proteins throughout the body and brain.

Liu-Ambrose concluded that the differences in the effects of both aerobic and strength training were small, but present. The all-inclusive effect is that any kind of exercise will improve cognitive function greatly. As with exercise for the body, it's best to incorporate aerobic and strength training for balanced fitness.

Exercise may increase midbrain size

The midbrain is used for reward learning, reinforcing behavior, and motivation. The result of an important and conclusive research study shows that physical exercise may increase midbrain size and improve brain function. The study was performed at the University of California Riverside by principal researcher Theodore Garland and a professor of biology.

The study took 20 years to complete, and the researchers looked at 65 generations of mice subjects. The mice were bred to have an increased desire to exercise and would voluntarily use the spin wheel in their cage more than regular mice. A comparison of the brain size of the exercising mice with the brain size of the regular mice showed that the mice that exercised had 13 percent greater volume in their midbrain size.

In past studies, using mammals and birds with naturally larger brains has shown a higher survival rate in adverse living situations. Also, the runner's high hormones produced within the brain after an intense workout have antidepressant effects, perhaps due to a drop in stress hormones.

Not too long ago, we needed these stress hormones to become sufficiently motivated to produce a fight or flight mechanism, which is a reaction that was necessary for human survival in centuries past. Now we produce the same hormones just by sitting at a desk talking with the boss. This is very likely to be the reason why exercising after a day at work feels so good.

Plus, a diet rich in omega 3 fatty acids, found in flaxseed and some fish, can be beneficial. These oils are believed to fill the spaces between brain neurons, thereby improving their exchange of electricity and functioning. These spaces between neurons may be wider due to heredity, or, drug or alcohol abuse, and can result in mood disorders.

Aside from understanding that physical exercise can increase midbrain size, there are specific brain activities that you can do to improve your brain dexterity, including reading, playing board games, crossword puzzles, and on the many Internet brain exercise sites, and bingo.

Brain workouts are especially good for improving the memory of older adults. The beneficial effects of these mind workouts can include improvements in memory, problem-solving ability, and mental clarity.

Just as you exercise your body to be healthier and function better, exercise for your brain may also help you think more clearly, more quickly, and yes, be smarter ... just think about it!

$$\text{🏃🏃}$$

Scrutinize your body with technology

Every day it seems that new wearable fitness gadgets and devices, that scrutinize your body and its reactions to exercise and your environment, appear on the market.

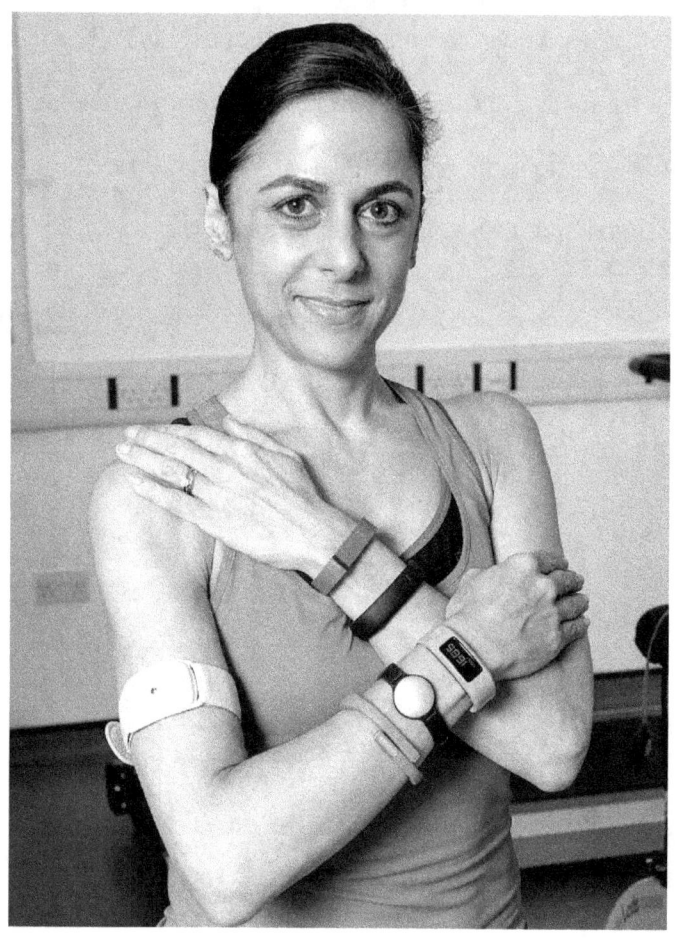

These interesting little computers can be very helpful in making your workouts more efficient, and more effective. They will measure your walking and running distances, your physical movements, and your body's physiological reactions, as you venture through your day. Some of them will even follow sleep patterns, and sleep depth, in order to wake you up at the optimal time accordingly. Then, the large amount of collected data can presented on their associated websites, in graphs and charts, for a better visual understanding.

The devices may have sensors that can be placed on your torso, on a wristband, your finger, or forehead. Many of these personal fitness devices make recommendations on:

- When to exercise
- How intensely to exercise, and when to speed up, or slow down
- What to eat, and how much
- When to get up off the couch, chair, or drivers seat, because you've been sitting too long
- The best time to wake up in the morning by sounding an alarm at the right time so you feel most rested. There's a gadget within your personal fitness device called an accelerometer, which closely monitors subtle movements and sounds like snoring, during the night.

These gadgets are great because by simply observing all the data, even for only one day, it can be like taking a lightning-fast crash course in getting to know your own body.

To get the most you can, pay very close attention to how you feel physically and emotionally as you acquire the data from activity to activity throughout your day. These devices offer a smarter way to help you get in shape, and can make the process easier, and more fun.

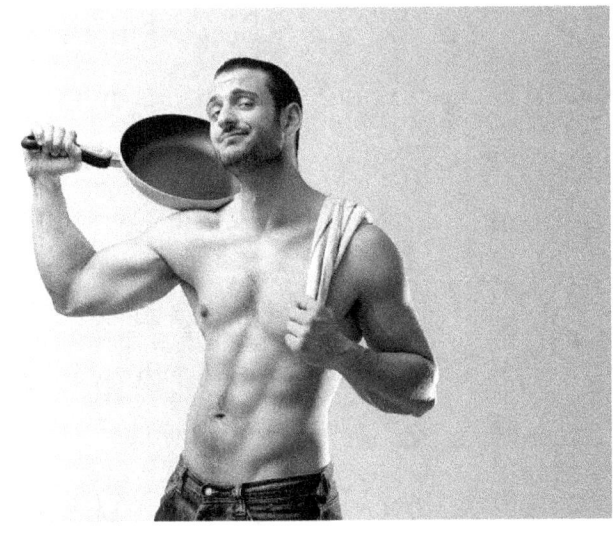

DIET

*F*ree your fridge

A great first step when you want to start eating better is to get rid of the temptations that may distract you from following healthier eating habits. When you're at that highly motivated point and you're ready to make big changes, it is time to toss out those unhealthy foods and free your fridge. Make room for fresh vegetables and fruit, whole grains, and lean protein sources.

Now that you've decided to eat better, it would be a smart move if you get junk foods and junk beverages out of your house so you're not tempted to snack during the day or night. Go ahead, clear it out, free your fridge, and restock it with healthier options.

But, you may be against throwing any food away and consider it to be wasteful. If so, you can eat that less nutritious food and gradually replace it with healthier alternatives.

Another option is to throw away half the unhealthy food all at once and then replace it with food that is more nutritious. In fact, for some people, a gradual change rather than a sudden switch that may be difficult to maintain is more likely to emerge as a new lifestyle that takes hold.

Then, if you're worried about getting hungry, keep healthy snacks on hand. Get low-calorie snack bars, bananas, or carrots and celery sticks (soaked in lightly salted water, left precut in the fridge in a container with water for quick access). In addition, you will now have room in your refrigerator to stock some low-fat/low-sugar yogurt and reduced-fat milk. Some great nonfat, low-calorie, and high-protein Greek yogurts are available.

One or two shelves in the fridge can be devoted to fresh fruit. If you find that you just cannot bear to rid your diet of sweets, then try keeping something low calorie on hand like peppermints or other small hard candy that you can suck on. Eating a few of these won't ruin your diet but will give you that little sugary fix you crave. Furthermore, many sugar-free candies are available, but beware, they are not always calorie free so you don't want to eat a lot of them.

If you want crunchies in your meals or snacks, then keep low-fat whole-wheat crackers on hand. Melba crackers are crunchy enough that they will likely satisfy, and they have very few calories. Another good food for satisfying your cravings for crunchies is low-fat microwave smaller serving popcorn.

Another great step to healthy eating when you're first starting the process is to take some time to learn about the foods that are the healthiest for you and how they operate within the body.

Most people understand that fruits, vegetables, low-fat meats, and low-fat dairy products are good for you, but not many people understand exactly what goes on in your body when you eat them.

A key is to learn about nutrients. When you understand how specific nutrients work and why you need them, you become more motivated to make healthier choices. Make use of Internet resources, books, movies, and cooking and nutrition classes. You'll find that education leads to motivation.

The USDA's guidelines for a healthy diet are based on real science and actual facts.

Are you struggling to figure out exactly what healthier eating is? There are many different kinds of diets, and it's difficult to determine which are effective and which are not. A great place to begin is by becoming familiar with the basic United States Department of Agriculture (USDA) guidelines for nutrition, which are based on facts and science:

- Increase vegetable and fruit intake, and eat a variety of vegetables, especially dark green, red, and orange veggies, beans, and peas.

- Consume at least half of all grains as whole grains, replacing refined grains.

- Moderate your intake of milk products, including yogurt, cheese, and soy beverages. When you do choose dairy foods, go for the fat-free or low-fat items. Low-fat Greek yogurt is, in fact, a high-quality protein source.

- Choose a variety of protein foods, including seafood, lean meat, poultry, eggs, beans, peas, soy products, and unsalted nuts and seeds.

- Increase the amount and variety of seafood consumed by choosing seafood in place of some meats and poultry.

- Replace protein foods that are higher in solid fats with foods that are lower in solid fats and calories. Use oils to replace solid fats where possible.

- Choose foods that provide more potassium, dietary fiber, calcium, and vitamin D, all of which may be lacking in American diets. These foods include vegetables, fruits, whole grains, milk, and milk products.

- Select an eating pattern at an appropriate calorie level that meets your nutrient needs over time.

Although basic in nature, these are a lot of recommendations to take in all at once. So that the changes you make will become part of your lifestyle gradually, and are not just a flash in the pan (humor intended), just read through the list and commit yourself to one change at a time. Commit to making that change permanent. Then you can make another change every couple of weeks, and so on.

For example, you may decide to eat one-half of your grains as whole grains for at least three weeks. You can also define different goals from those listed above. It's your choice. It may take a few weeks (or longer) before the changes you make become easier to maintain.

You will begin to feel the satisfaction of small successes as you make healthier nutrition choices. You will have more energy for exercise and you'll have smoother skin, clearer eyes, and many other positive results.

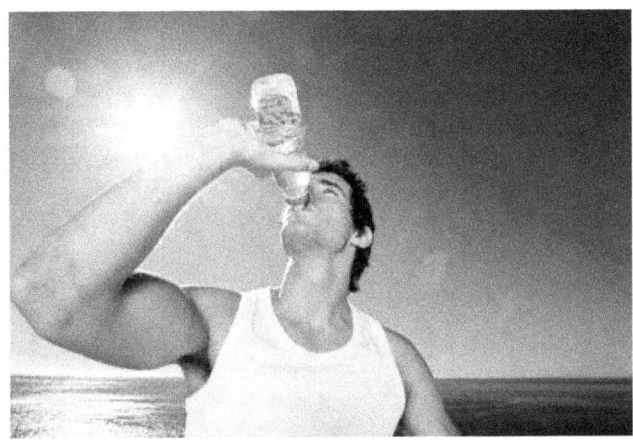

*T*he world's four healthiest beverages

Water:

Water is the best beverage of all, which is confirmed by the fact that all the other healthiest beverages are mostly water. Our body is 70% to 80% water. On the occasions that you want just a plain glass of water, you want it to be high-quality, clean, and clear water. Some people drink tap water and in some cities the tap water is very pure, and delicious.

The way you'll know that your tap water is of good quality is to seek out its quality report – you will probably find the report for your locale on the Internet. If you get water from your own well, have it tested by a water testing lab for bacteria and other potential problems. A technician can take a sample back to the lab and check it out. A simpler and free way to test your water is to smell it and taste it.

Sure, oceans of water exist all over the planet, and it may seem silly to pay for water. Even so, you probably want your body to be made of mostly pure, clean, and healthy water. The rule of "eight 8-oz. glasses of water a day" is a good approximation, but note that this is for the average-size person. Your daily water need will vary depending on your body weight, activity level, and how hot and dry it is where you live.

Vegetable juices:

Many of us are always looking for more ways to add veggies to our diet. It's not easy to get the USDA-recommended three to five servings of vegetables every day. Fresh vegetable juice helps meet this goal. Especially nutritious are beet, tomato, spinach, and kale juices.

Green tea:

Green tea has beneficial phytonutrients and lower levels of caffeine than other teas. With increasing research on green tea, more health benefits are being found. A cancer fighter, green tea has antioxidant effects that lower the risk of conditions ranging from bacterial or viral infections to cardiovascular disease, cancer, stroke, periodontal disease, and osteoporosis.

Fortified bottled water:

Containing vitamins and naturally sweetened fruit juices, some fortified bottled waters offer a full day's supply of vitamin C while others promise no artificial sweeteners and a nice, fruity taste. If it helps you drink more water, do it.

*P*owerfully addictive HFCS

Have you ever indulged in a sweet dessert that made you think you might never be able to get enough of it? Well, it's likely that it was made with powerfully addictive high-fructose corn syrup (HFCS), which is frequently found in soda pop, ice cream, crackers, cereal, and many fat-free processed foods, and the list goes on.

The term "high-fructose corn syrup" sounds healthy enough to the uninformed consumer, but although fructose and corn may be healthy, in the case of high-fructose corn syrup they're not. HFCS is a high-calorie, high-carbohydrate sweetener that has no nutritional value.

HFCS has been chemically altered in a way that just so happens to shut down your brain's production of leptin, a fat-regulating hormone that lets you know when you've had enough to eat. Leptin sends signals from your brain to your stomach saying, "I'm satisfied and satiated," and your hunger diminishes. When you start reading more food labels as part of your healthier lifestyle, you may be amazed at how many food products have HFCS in them.

On American food labels, the ingredients are listed in order by the amount of an ingredient in the product, from most to least. In other words, the ingredients at the top of the list on the label are what the product is mostly made of. If you see HFCS on the list, especially if it's in the top few ingredients, then it's a food you would do well to eat sparingly if at all.

Choosing foods that don't contain any HFCS is best. Just recently, the Food and Drug Administration (FDA) approved a few great new sugar alternatives:

The new zero or low-calorie sweeteners like Truvia, Z-Sweet, and Sun Crystals are made from natural sources such as erythritol and stevia. You can find these sweeteners in most grocery stores. In addition to their obvious use in cold drinks, you can also use these natural sweeteners to replace sugars in hot beverages, on oatmeal, and even in some baked foods.

A popular no-calorie sweetener is stevia rebaudiana. It's a leaf that has been used all over the world for years as a safe, natural, no-calorie sweetener. You can find stevia under the names PureVia, SweetLeaf, and sometimes mixed with erythritol in Truvia.

Erythritol is an all-natural zero-calorie sweetener fermented from the natural sugars found in many fruits and vegetables. It has zero calories. Some popular low-calorie alcohol-based sweeteners include Sorbitol, Xylitol, and Maltitol.

It would be great not to overuse any sweetener at all so that your body eventually learns that it doesn't need sweet foods to be satisfied. It's important to remember that sugar isn't bad for you, just like all fats aren't terrible for you. In their proper forms, sugars and fats can be a healthy part of any wholesome diet.

🏃‍♂️

*T*he fastest rate that you can lose weight safely

If you've decided to lose weight, instead of going on a crash diet to lose a lot of weight quickly, you need to understand that the fastest rate to lose weight safely is one pound a week. Don't flinch because that sounds too slow, because if you lose one pound a week, that equals a total of 52 pounds per year. And at that rate it's more likely you'll be gradually making lifestyle changes that will stick. So that your new lifestyle will support the weight you lose, and permanently.

So, if you want to lose 10 pounds, give yourself at least 10 weeks. You'll be more likely to keep the weight off if you give yourself the time to make and maintain necessary dietary and lifestyle changes. Plus, the body weight that you lose will be mostly body fat, With slower weight loss, you'll be less prone to losing body muscle.

With a crash diet, you're more likely to lose muscle, which over time slows your metabolism. After an extreme crash diet, it's easy to fall right back into old eating habits and gain even more weight due to a slower metabolism. To determine a proper weight-loss goal, it helps to make sure your goal is:

1. Reasonable

2. Measurable

3. Attainable

Your first nutrition or fitness goal following these parameters may be as simple as replacing one soda a day with a glass of water. This will reduce your caloric intake, and even if you drink no-calorie soda pop, it's better for your body to choose water instead.

If you eat fast foods for lunch, replace those foods with a nutritious healthy lunch from home every other day. Try this for one month. This nutritional goal is reasonable, measurable, and attainable. You may find that healthier lunches from home taste better and help you feel your best.

When you start by taking small steps, you are not cutting out the foods you are used to all at once. By taking time to learn about your eating habits and slowly replacing less nutritious foods with healthier alternatives, you will begin to feel better physically, mentally, and emotionally, plus, the changes are more likely to stick.

Make one change toward better nutrition at a time and then all the small nutritional changes and fitness goals you've attained will add up.

犭身

*I*s *childhood obesity genetic?*

We have an epidemic of childhood obesity in America, but why? There are no simple answers, and each child's situation is different. Many distinct factors must be considered. The ongoing discussion of nature vs. nurture might make some people believe that certain children are naturally doomed to being overweight because of a genetic predisposition. Formal study, plus ongoing anecdotal reports show that this is simply *not* the case. The epidemic of childhood obesity in America is being caused by lifestyle. The epidemic of childhood obesity in America is caused by how the children are being nurtured.

According to the American Obesity Association, childhood obesity is the result of a combination of lack of physical activity and poor eating habits, both of which can be changed. These are some of the factors contributing to childhood obesity:

- Generations before the obesity epidemic, children spent their time playing sports, riding bikes, running, and jumping. Today the average kid spends his or her time very differently, indoors playing video games, watching TV, or spending time on the computer.

- Children develop poor eating habits by eating high-calorie foods and super-sized fast food items even when they are not hungry.

- Children may be exposed to unhealthy and excessive eating in the home.

- An unhealthy at-home lifestyle may directly influence the child's lifestyle habits and can lead to a lifetime of poor nutrition and inactivity.

The best way to combat the obesity epidemic is to help children learn a healthier lifestyle as they grow and develop. On a nationwide level, many schools are beginning to encourage active and healthy lifestyles by removing soda and candy machines from hallways and providing USDA-approved school lunches.

In addition, the National Task Force on Childhood Obesity is helping to pave the way. A helpful tool that can be found at the USDA website is the *Choose My Plate* program, an excellent source of basic information and advice on healthy eating habits.

There is no instant cure for childhood obesity. Most medical, fitness, and nutrition professionals believe that the solution is to be found by addressing the root cause of lifestyle choices at home and at school. The goal of the Task Force on Childhood Obesity is to solve America's problem of childhood obesity within a generation.

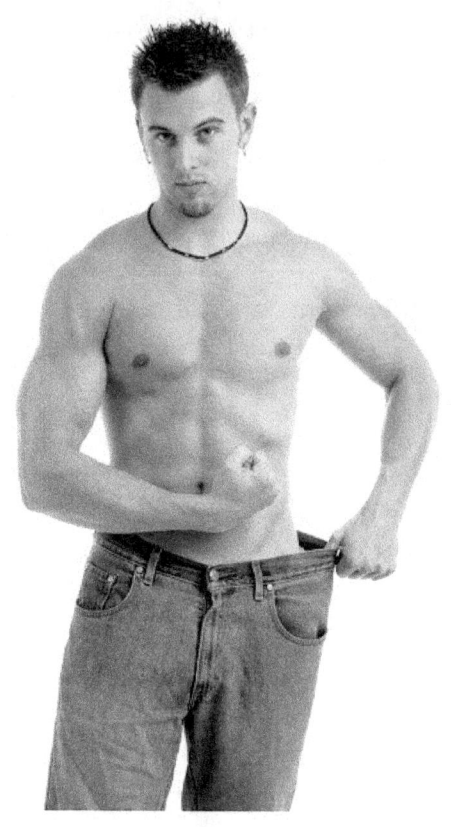

*T*he truth concerning your body weight

You may have become discouraged if you've been unsuccessful with past attempts to manage body weight. You may be self-conscious because you believe that people think less of you because you are overweight, but you are not alone. The truth of the matter on body weight regulation is that Americans are overeating.

In the U.S. portion sizes are often double what they should be. Usually people who are at their best body weight are eating reasonable portion sizes of whatever diet they choose.

*T*hree great lifestyle habits

These three great lifestyle habits will help you reach and then maintain your ideal body weight:

1) Healthier eating consistently.

Many healthy diet plans are available, and a lot of them are great. The best of the diets actually have a few key elements in common. They include a wide variety of foods that are plant based, they emphasize exercise, plus, discuss the psychological component of weight loss.

Some diets have evolved over centuries, in particular in regions across the world where there is easy access to nutritious food and a natural need for physical activity built into the lifestyle. Some of these cultures are naturally very healthy, and are people who manage their body weight well. Greece, France, Italy, and Japan are just a few of these cultures worth naming. They all have access to healthy food and live an active lifestyle naturally.

2) Exercise.

To put it simply ... get moving. Somehow as Americans we have developed a tendency to promote inactivity in our lifestyle. Great cars, video games, movies, and computers all contribute to our physical inactivity.

In the media, we are always being encouraged to join a gym or buy a diet book, and many well-intentioned Americans do these things, but soon find themselves losing motivation. Unfortunately, the American lifestyle, by nature, does not encourage sufficient physical activity to maintain a healthy level of fitness.

If motivation is part of your difficulty, then looking for outside support may be a useful approach. Tell your friends and family about your intentions to be more physically active, and ask them to support you in your endeavor or, better yet, get them to join you!

Numerous Internet groups can offer support as well, some free and some commercial. The Weight Watchers program continues to have a very good success rate partly due to the support groups and regular meetings that it promotes. Another highly recommended free website and smartphone app is MyFitnessPal.com, which is also a portal to numerous additional useful fitness apps.

3) Continually increase your knowledge of nutrition.

The body is a complex machine and it takes some of the fuel and nutrients that you consume and stores them for later. Therefore, it is important to know that you are supplying your body with all the vital nutrients that it needs, and in proper amounts.

Obvious, but worth mentioning, is that one of the best ways to know which foods are optimal for you is to simply read up on nutrition. In terms of eating well and exercising effectively, knowledge is power. Keep reading about nutrition, and continue to learn about what your body needs to be healthy.

As we get older, it's more important than ever to eat a diet high in nutrition, and to maintain a healthy body weight. And once you reach your ideal body weight, and you will, compared to the challenge of losing weight, maintaining it is pretty easy by:

1) Healthier eating consistently.

2) Exercise

3) Continually increase your knowledge of nutrition.

*A*n apple a day... here's why

There's no easier way to get a big dose of nutrition, than eating an apple. In all likelihood, you first experienced the apple's delightful flavor when you were a baby, and were fed applesauce, maybe as your original real food.

Whether it's a Granny Smith, a McIntosh, or a Red Delicious raw or in a pie, you probably think of the apple as an old friend. What they say about apples is true; one a day is a quick way to live better… here's why.

Apples are grown all over the world these days, so they're always in season. Apples are high in fiber, vitamins, minerals, and antioxidants. They're fat free, cholesterol free, and low in sodium. In other words, eating apples, as few as one a day, is a smart part of your healthy lifestyle.

An apple a day cuts your risk of heart disease. Sometimes it's hard to remember which foods are effective for which parts of your body. An apple is shaped a bit like a heart so remember that apples are good for your heart.

It's the magnesium and potassium in apples that help regulate your blood pressure and keep your heart beating steadily. It's the flavonoid quercetin, a naturally occurring antioxidant that protects your artery walls from damage and keeps your blood flowing smoothly. In fact, adding flavonoid-rich foods like apples to your diet has been scientifically confirmed to lower your risk of heart disease.

The next time you pick up an apple, to get the most

from it, examine it carefully, think about where it was grown, mindfully thank the person who picked it, and acknowledge how it was delivered to you. Think about its nutrients, and remember that "an apple a day may indeed keep the doctor away".

妰妰

Super hero nuts and grains

Divided into subgroups, what follows is a list of super hero nuts and grains that are undoubtedly favored by our favorite idols to keep our city safe from crime and dinosaurs.

Whole-grain bread, pasta, and brown rice:

The first thing you can check when purchasing bread or pasta is 100% whole grain or not. Check the list of ingredients looking for the exact term "100% whole-wheat flour" as one of the first ingredients listed. Wheat bran is a cancer-fighting grain that also helps us regulate good digestion.

Brown rice is a better choice than refined white rice for the same reason that choosing whole-wheat bread over white bread is better. Whole-wheat flour or brown rice that is turned into white flour or white rice actually loses some of the vitamin B3, vitamin B1, vitamin B6, manganese, phosphorus, and iron, all the dietary fiber, and many essential fatty acids.

Even when processed white rice (or processed white flour) is said to be enriched, it is not in the same form as the original unprocessed food. Just as with vegetables and fruits, grain is best eaten with the fibrous outer coating whenever possible.

While beans are rich in certain essential amino acids, brown rice is rich in other essential amino acids. So, the combination of rice and beans makes a high-quality complete protein. Whenever possible, mix some beans into your rice, or some rice in with your beans. Bean chili, for example, is especially nutritious and delicious with brown rice added.

Seeds:

Quinoa is the seed of the goosefoot plant. It is a pseudo cereal, not an actual cereal or grain. Quinoa is closely related to beetroots, spinach, and tumbleweeds. Even so, the nutrient composition of quinoa is better than that of cereals. Quinoa seeds contain essential amino acids like lysine, lots of calcium, phosphorus, and iron.

Amaranth is also considered a pseudo cereal. It's a good source of protein and amaranth is especially packed with the essential amino acid lysine. Grains like wheat and corn are rich in the amino acids that amaranth lacks, so amaranth mixed with other grains is a healthy combination.

Almonds and walnuts:

These nuts are packed with omega 3 fats. These are the healthier of the nuts and will provide many health benefits, including cardiovascular protection, better cognitive function, and anti-inflammatory advantages relating to asthma, rheumatoid arthritis, and inflammatory skin diseases like eczema and psoriasis, plus, support the immune system.

Beans and lentils:

While black beans are a good source of fiber that can

lower cholesterol, so are lentils. The high-fiber content of black beans and lentils helps to maintain blood sugar levels.

See if you can find a multi-bean mix at the store that includes lentils and black beans, navy beans, pinto beans, red beans, and kidney beans and then combine it with some rice for a real power-food, complete-protein meal. Consider making a delicious soup or chili, hot or cold, with the addition of tomatoes, onions, garlic, and your favorite spices.

It's not commonly known, but green peas are a nutritious source of complete protein. Whether you get your peas in pea soup, whole and in a bowl, or pea protein powder.

*M*eals in a rush

So you've eaten a healthy breakfast of oatmeal, whole-wheat cereal, or whole-grain toast, you've avoided fat and sugar and included some fresh fruit. Now, as you anticipate your day of continued healthier eating, plan ahead to avoid eating meals in a rush.

If you often eat in a hurry and at odd times of the day, you're probably inclined to rush for a meal which may not be as nutritious and healthy as you would like. Planning ahead for these times actually works. Instead of grabbing a fast food lunch on the run it helps to plan in advance to take a bagged nutritious lunch from home. Remember to include some fresh fruit and vegetables, usually the more colorful they are, the healthier they are.

If fast food is all you have time for, then try to choose the fast food restaurants that are healthier. You can buy sandwiches to order at some fast food places, and some grocery delicatessens often have pre-made nutritious sandwiches.

Some fast food places make most of their food without frying, like Subway, for example, and some have a good amount of fresh veggies. Many old-time fast food restaurants, like McDonald's and Burger King, offer some healthier choices these days all-be-it not their most advertised.

Then there's dinner, having a simple plan before you get home is smart, but with a fast-paced lifestyle, sometimes making healthier dinner choices is difficult. One way that may solve this problem is to plan your evening meals for the week just before you do the weekly shopping. Be cautious, don't go to the grocery store when you're hungry because you're more likely to buy junk food and generally more food than you need.

Eventually, you want your meals to be based on fresh vegetables and fruits. Almost every meal should also include a low-fat protein source like fish, boneless and skinless poultry, or brown rice combined with beans. When combined, rice and beans have all the important amino acids to constitute a complete protein. Because protein is digested slowly, it's best to have some with most meals so that you are less likely to get hungry and make poor choices between meals.

Nutrition is at the core of living your best and creating your best self possible. As you manage your healthy diet and nutrition plan, the additional components of fitness will fall into place more naturally. You'll have more energy for exercise and better stress control, good sleep hygiene, and an overall higher quality of life.

🏃🏃

Know your fats

An important part of your healthier lifestyle is to know all you can about your dietary fats. To begin, know that the USDA recommends that fat intake be between 20% and 35% of total calories for adults. The recommendations from the USDA are based on real science and actual facts, and many fad diets are not.

You may already know that the healthiest fats are the unsaturated type. In general, nuts, vegetable oils, and fish are sources of unsaturated fats and they can help lower cholesterol, and assist in your body's use of vitamins A, E, D, and K.

Fats to avoid are the saturated and transfats types

found in fried foods, fatty meats, butter, and margarine, including fats that are partially hydrogenated. It's best to avoid these fats altogether.

The fat-free diets of the past are an unhealthy approach to weight loss because some fats are necessary in your diet. Be aware that foods advertised as fat free are often high in sugars and calories.

Packaged foods are required to have their nutritional information on the label, and most restaurants are required to give you a list of ingredients, nutrient types, and calories if you request it. Nevertheless, in many situations, like a meal in a restaurant, you'll have to estimate a food's nutrition.

When it comes to dietary fat, remember that a healthy target is approximately 15% to 25% of your total calories from fat. To determine the percentage of calories from fat of any food that has a food label, divide the total calories from fat (say, 25) by the total number of calories (e.g., 100). In this case, 25 divided by 100 equals 0.25% (the same as 25%).

Also, the approximation of fat intake can be spread

throughout your day as well. For instance, you might have a burger for lunch and then to make up for it have a salad for dinner. In both of these situations you'll have to make nutritional estimations because these foods aren't necessarily labeled.

Using estimations, when these two meals are combined, you might average 23% of calories from fat. This means that you don't need to worry about having that one burger because your average fat percentage for the combination of foods at the end of that day is 23%.

Don't try to average more than one day at a time because wider dietary fat variations may disrupt your body's ability to utilize fat, as well as your metabolism.

What about weight loss and weight gain? On any given day, if you eat more total calories than you burn, some of those extra calories will be stored as body fat. If you burn more calories than you eat, you'll experience weight loss.

You can abide by the general rule of thumb regarding calories in versus calories out. Choose a wide variety of nutritious foods, lean proteins, colorful vegetables and fruits, plus, healthy fats.

Another important factor is that with more exercise your metabolism (the body's rate of burning calories) speeds up, so if you exercise consistently, even while you sleep you are burning more calories. If you don't get enough physical activity, and you eat a diet high in calories, you'll gain weight.

While it's very much about the simple calories in versus calories out principle, genetics, age, and gender also play a part in the weight-gain formula. Some people need to diet and exercise a little more than others. For everyone, consistency is key!

*A*re you burning up your muscles?

When you diet and exercise to lose weight, it's important to make sure that you are reducing body fat but maintaining body muscle. When you restrict the calories in your diet, there is a good chance that you may lose body muscle along with body fat.

The danger of burning up your muscles is especially present if you're losing weight quickly, as with crash diets. Most health and fitness experts agree that the safest amount of weight to lose is about one pound a week.

With a crash diet, it's possible that you're losing some body muscle along with body fat. Then having lost body muscle, it's likely that you'll gain back more body fat. Crash diets don't allow for enough time to learn the new lifestyle habits that are necessary.

A decrease in body muscle will mean a slowing of your metabolism. It's your body's muscle that keeps your metabolism higher during the day and night – burning calories 24/7.

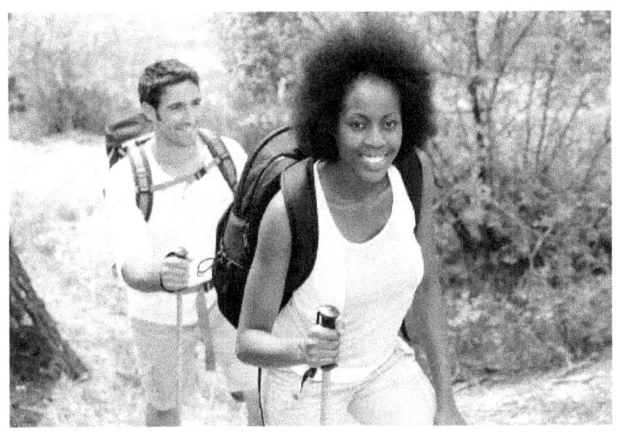

WELLNESS

How to fully participate in your life

It's possible that a person who doesn't eat right, and doesn't exercise, may have and long life anyway. Nevertheless, many of us have decided to bank on being fitter by eating right and exercising regularly. Besides the increased likelihood of living longer, physical fitness will also improve the ability to fully participate in life also. By making our senses sharper, our thinking clearer, and giving us the best energy and vitality, physical fitness.

Exercising and eating right is not always easy, but we know that the payoff is well worth the investment.

Better overall health allows us greater feelings of pleasure, quicker thinking, a more satisfying sex life, healthier skin, and oomph for more time to share with friends and family.

$$\dot{\tilde{\lambda}}\tilde{\eth}$$

*H*ow you can better almost immediately!

Exercising outdoors is the best thing you can do to help you look better almost immediately. Depending on your athletic ability, 20 or more minutes of moderate outside exercise three to five days evenly spaced throughout the week is all you need to look better right away, even the very first day. Activities such as brisk walking, biking, or jogging are most likely to do the trick.

This outdoor moderate-intensity exercise is invigorating for the whole body, your muscles, skin, heart, and lungs, and gives you a good dose of fresh air and sunlight. Listen to your favorite music, just enjoy yourself. You'll be invigorated - full of smiles for the rest of the day.

Could your body be a lemon?

While some people have a natural talent for physical performance, some find it more exigent. If you think you were born into a body that's a lemon, you're probably incorrect. But, even for any special challenges you face there are solutions. With consistent adherence to a well put together fitness program, you can make dramatic changes in your athletic performance, how you look, and how you feel. Even if your challenge is a handicap or illness, a good diet and exercise program can have great effects on your overall wellness.

The key to increasing your level of fitness and maintaining a healthy weight is exercise and diet consistency. Gradually over time, your body's shape and size develop largely as a result of how you eat and exercise.

Other factors like genetics, your natural energy level, and inherited physical prowess certainly play a role, but a lack of these natural abilities can be overcome with a solid fitness program and healthy lifestyle. If you think your body is a lemon, even if you've inherited poor health, fitness helps.

The body adapts to whatever challenges you create for it and the changes contribute to your overall fitness level. For example, if you are consistently performing resistance exercises with more weight than you used previously, then your muscles will grow to adapt to the new greater challenge. Your muscles will become bigger and stronger to adapt to lifting those heavier weights.

If you require greater cardiovascular demands of your body by exercising, your lungs will learn to process oxygen more efficiently, and your heart will become stronger from the increased demands.

Consistently and gradually making increasing demands of your body creates a change in your body's physical ability so that it's better able to respond to the greater demands. You will change the body you've

inherited as you become more fit. It's these changes —
performed consistently — that are the key to success in
achieving and maintaining a higher level of fitness. Got
lemons? Make lemonade.

*E*xergaming is a gateway to fitness

The Internet, video gaming while sitting, and TV
have made it far too easy for many of us to sit still.
Children and adolescents are especially likely to spend
many hours each day doing these and other sedentary
activities, when the children of previous decades were
running and jumping.

However, technology is not entirely to blame for our
sedentary lifestyle, and in fact, there is a particular
technology that may actually help, and it's called
exergaming. It's proving to be that, in many cases,
exergaming is a gateway to fitness!

Exergames are basically physically interactive video games. As the participant plays the exergame, the movements of the characters on the screen interact with the participant playing the game in a way that exercising his or her body. For example, a player can be holding an imitation tennis racket, baseball bat, or golf club, and as the player moves to perform an activity, the pseudo player on the screen displays corresponding moves.

So, instead of lying on the sofa, the player is jumping, swinging, reaching, and sweating in active participation, while enjoying the benefits of technology and the amazing games.

That exergaming is beneficial seems obvious, and it's supported by a lot of clinical research. As exergames become more sophisticated, we can safely predict that they can help reduce the time children are sedentary and get them up and moving.

It may even help children and adolescents realize which physical activities and sports they may really enjoy, which in turn might provide a gateway into an active lifestyle.

If people like exergaming, they are more likely to play the games consistently, and remember that consistency is the key to any progress in fitness level. If you're used to sitting and not moving, then getting up is a great first step, and activities like exergaming can make for infinite progress.

Potential benefits of exergaming include:

- You can begin to reduce the amount of time you spend being sedentary.

- It's a great steppingstone to help kids explore the type of physical activity they really enjoy and are good at.

- It can even increase their confidence to try something outside the world of exergaming like tennis on a real court or golfing on an actual course.

- It can help with your exercise adherence. Many people quit exercise programs because they become bored or do not see results quickly enough.

Exergaming can be a great alternative on one of those

days when you just don't feel like exercising or you just don't have the time to go to the gym or the park. Exergaming can give you another option for training and exercise.

*E*xercise is the magic pill

"Exercise is the magic pill," says Michael R. Bracko, education chairman of the American College of Sports Medicine's Consumer Information Committee. "Exercise can even cure some forms of diseases heart disease and diabetes." A weak heart may be strengthened by cardiovascular exercise, with a good diet type II diabetes can be greatly improved.

Exercise has been implicated in helping people prevent or recover from some forms of cancer. Exercise can help reduce the pain and swelling of some forms of arthritis.

Exercise can even play an important role in the management of depression. Many seasoned exercisers and fitness professionals say that "exercise is the elixir of life."

*W**earable fitness gadgets*

You can learn a lot about your body very quickly by wearing a fitness-monitoring gadget. Usually worn on the wrist, chest, or fingertip, they allow you to follow just how your body responds to your daily activities, including exercise and sleep.

At the very least, the data collected may give you the extra motivation that you've been wanting. Here's a list of wearable fitness gadgets' important features:

- It's comfortable to wear 24/7.

- It has a battery that lasts four days or more.

- It gives very specific information.

- It tells you specifically what to do.

- It tracks daily and sleep data.

- It can upload data online and presents it to you in a way that's easy to understand and to utilize.

It used to take lots and lots of exercise sessions to learn as much as you can by using one of these devices for a couple of days. A personal fitness gadget is likely to reduce the time it takes to get to know how your body responds to exercise. These gadgets can also increase the efficiency of your workouts, the effectiveness, and safety.

A variety of wearable personal-fitness monitoring devices is available today, but this is only the beginning. More recently developed gadgets have sensors like an optical scanner to track blood flow and heart rate. Another feature of some devices is a sweat monitor that compares skin temperature to outside-the-body temperature.

Many wearable fitness gadgets also measure calories burned, number of steps taken, resting average heart rate, and depth of sleep. Some can even wake you up at the most favorable time in regard to your sleep rhythms.

T*he weight-loss formula is simple*

If you have struggled to maintain a healthy body weight, then you may have come to realize that being overweight is a lot more complicated than just overeating. It's best to begin your program with the understanding that you must combine exercise with diet to achieve weight loss. The weight-loss formula is plain and simple: Exercise plus diet equals weight loss.

A healthy and calorie-appropriate diet must be combined with regular exercise, and both must be included in your daily fitness program consistently to achieve weight loss. If on any given day you eat more calories than you burn, some of those extra calories will be stored as body fat. If instead, on that same day, you had burned more calories exercising than the calories that you consumed, then you would lose weight.

In other words, people who don't get enough physical activity and who eat a diet high in calories are going to gain weight, plain and simple. Exercising, ideally, 150 minutes a week with at least some exercise almost every day is recommended. This not only burns calories when you perform the exercise, but your metabolism speeds up so that your body burns more calories, for the rest of the day, and maybe even for days to follow.

Exercise combined with diet is the true key to the long-term maintenance of your healthy body weight. Dietitians, fitness pros, and wellness experts agree that the healthiest diet is one that is plant based.

Proteins should represent less than one-quarter of your plate. The protein group was once known as the meat group, but over time it has transitioned to incorporate other protein-rich foods such as fish, shellfish, poultry, eggs, beans, peas, nuts, seeds, and certain dairy products like low-fat milk and yogurt.

Sugars and simple carbohydrates should also represent less than one-quarter of your plate. The remainder of your plate is then left for colorful fruits and vegetables. Again, the healthiest diet is one that is plant based.

If you are just beginning your quest for fitness, it's best to be easy on yourself. Rather than expecting to adhere to these recommendations perfectly, start with a comfortable level of intensity for both exercise and diet. It's important to note that people progress at different rates and that genetics, age, and gender play a part in the weight gain or loss formula.

Try changing one thing each week, such as exercising almost every other day, decrease your meal portion sizes, or, increase the amount of colorful fruits and vegetables in your diet. Then, in a few weeks, you can increase the intensity and frequency of your exercise.

And in a few months, you'll begin to feel that your body is tightening up and that you have more energy than you did in the past – you are improving your level of fitness.

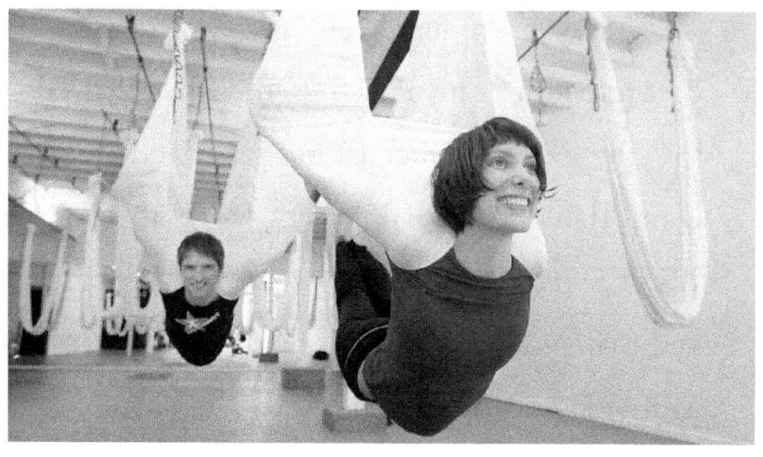

Do you find working out boring?

If you need to add exercise to your wellness plan but find working out boring, then try looking for something that you might consider extraordinary. Something as simple as changing your routine on a regular basis, so it actually never does become routine, may be all you need to stimulate your enthusiasm.

If you attend exercise classes, you know that every class instructor has his or her own unique techniques and approach. When you vary instructors, you'll probably enjoy the diversity.

It may also be especially interesting if you look for a class leader who's new to the facility. And, why not try an extraordinary class like pole dancing, ViPR, Tabata, or Unnata Aerial Yoga.

An intriguing favorite is the New York City-based Unnata Aerial Yoga, which combines traditional yoga with the physical training of an aerial acrobat. Unnata Aerial Yoga involves adapting common yoga poses to an off-the-ground position – it's a lot of fun!

In Unnata Aerial Yoga, the student is supported off the floor by a soft, fabric trapeze. The lack of limitations allows one's yoga practice to creatively adapt and the practitioner to learn new movements. Developed for all experience levels, no aerial, acrobatic, or yoga experience is needed. You're off the ground and free from that pesky gravity.

*S*mall steps

Before you go out and break your back trying to get in some hardcore exercise, relax and develop a workout that you might truly stick with and even enjoy. After all, if you enjoy the day's exercise session, you are more likely to want to repeat it. So be sure to perform your exercise activities at an intensity that is comfortable for you and not too painful.

Whether you like to train at a very high level of intensity, or, if you prefer moderate or even low intensity exercise, in order to achieve what you're working for will be better and safer when you take small steps.

As a lower intensity exerciser, you might choose daily activities that provide accidental exercise, for example, parking at the far end of the parking lot then walking, or taking the stairs instead of the escalator or elevator.

If you were to move from a one-story home into a two-story home, the additional exercise climbing the stairs may burn enough calories to lose ten pounds over the course of a year. It's these and other seemingly insignificant choices, made on a regular basis, that will make a big difference toward your long-term fitness goals.

FAVORITE DIETS, BOOKS, AND APPS

A *Full Life Without Dieting*

The celebrated bariatric surgeon Michael Snyder's book is titled *A Full Life without Dieting* and it offers an insider's perspective on weight loss. He advocates rejecting the diet mentality that thrives on restrictions, deprivations, and total reversals of lifestyle.

Using the science of fullness and introducing a new definition of healthy, in *A Full Life without Dieting,* Dr. Snyder brings us weight-control strategies that are rooted in our physiology and proves that the narcotic effect of fullness is the ultimate weapon in the battle for weight loss. Snyder provides industry insider tips, tools, and information that have helped countless patients succeed in their weight-loss efforts. The reader will learn how to:

- Choose from a variety of practical strategies to achieve sustainable weight loss regardless of dietary habits and preferences.

- End the confusion over portion control by synching visual and physiological cues of fullness.

- Be full with less food, but equally as satisfied (if not more so!).

- Apply a cheat prescription so you can still say yes to indulgences and temptations without feeling like a failure.

- Take advantage of the five intentional steps of digestion to gain effortless control of your dietary behavior.

- Find fulfillment in a physical activity that is inexpensive, easy, and convenient.

With these strategies and definitions, you can move from persistent dieting to living true to yourself and from being

unhappily overweight. You can learn to become a

healthy individual who recognizes a happy weight better than a scale does.

Dr. Snyder knows it's not the surgery that creates success in his patients, it's what they do afterward that counts. It is from this rich body of experience and practical wisdom that he's created these strategies to help you lose 10, 20, 30, 50 pounds—or more!

*Y*our Body Is Your Gym

Author Mark Lauren describes a simple exercise program that has proven to be very effective for many. It teaches the reader how to do a complete workout using only the weight of his or her body. It offers three levels of ability, so it will match any fitness level. Mark Lauren is a physical trainer of the troops in U.S. Special Operations. His book shows an ingeniously simple, do-anywhere program for getting into amazing shape.

Special Operations military forces are often on the front lines, and Mark Lauren has prepared nearly 1,000 troops by getting them leaner and stronger quickly. The *You Are Your Own Gym* program is composed of simple exercises that require nothing more than the resistance of your own body weight and these exercises can help you reach a higher level of fitness by simultaneously improving balance and agility.

Armed with Mark Lauren's motivation techniques, expert training, and nutrition advice, you'll see rapid results by working out just 30 minutes a day four times a week, whether in your living room, yard, garage, hotel room, or office. Lauren's exercises build more metabolism-enhancing muscle than weight lifting, burn more body fat calories than aerobics, and are safer than both.

To get started, choose your workout level:

1. Basic
2. First class
3. Master class
4. Chief class

Then, all you have to do is follow the clear instructions for 125 exercises that work every muscle from your neck to your ankles. Forget about gym memberships, free weights, and infomercial contraptions. You need to rely on only one thing, your own body.

🏃

*B*ob Greene's *The Best Life Diet*

From the best-selling author of *Get With The Program* and *Bob Greene's Total Body Makeover* comes *The Best Life Diet,* which is a lifetime plan for losing weight and keeping it off. Bob Greene's book helped Oprah achieve her dramatic weight loss, and he can help you too.

You'll eat the same delicious food that Oprah enjoys, and just like Oprah, you'll have Bob's good advice with you at every step. Unlike a celebrity, however, you don't need to hire a staff of experts to aid and advise you. Bob's plan can be easily tailored to an array of tastes, lifestyles, and activity levels and will act as your personal trainer and private nutritionist. Just open the book and let Bob help you get started down the path toward your best possible life.

What sets Bob apart from all the other experts who claim to have plans that work is that he admits that weight loss is very difficult. Seventeen years of watching people struggle to lose weight on a seemingly endless string of trendy crash diets only to backslide and regain the pounds they shed, plus, more has taught Bob that dropping pounds is a complex combination of many factors.

By acknowledging that being overweight is not the result of simple laziness, but a complicated web of social rituals, cultural expectations, and habits that drive people to gain weight, Greene attacks the problem of weight loss realistically and offers not a short-lived quick-fix formula, but a long-term program that accounts for the challenges and constraints of the real world.

Divided into three phases *The Best Life Diet* gives you the tools you need to change your life. In each phase, you'll be asked to reexamine the decisions you make daily and gradually alter your habits to achieve lasting results. The book also includes easy to follow meal plans that make it simple to meet your daily energy and nutrient requirements, whether you are on the run and breakfast means a quick smoothie or you have time to shop for fresh produce and make something special.

Most importantly, Bob's plan doesn't end once you've lost the weight. Instead, it gives you the tools you need to make living your best life second nature because, for Greene, a diet is not something you go on or off, but a set of guidelines that help you claim the life you deserve.

The Volumetrics Diet

The Volumetrics Diet offers a time-tested and effective well-balanced diet with no banned foods. Exercise is an important component and *The Volumetrics Diet* contributes many positive reviews by professionals within the health and fitness industry.

The Volumetrics Diet lays out a commonsense eating plan. It empowers readers to replace on-and-off dieting with a healthier lifestyle that includes low-calorie and nutritious foods and regular and consistent exercise.

The Volumetrics Diet plan looks at the energy density of foods. According to Dr. Rolls, awareness of the energy density of food (the number of calories in a specific volume of food) is the key to achieving healthy, long-term weight loss. Dieters are encouraged to eat low-calorie bulkier foods that are more filling so they feel full and satisfied after consuming fewer calories.

Volumetrics relies on foods with low energy density and high water content such as fruits and vegetables. Dr. Rolls believes that by eating low-calorie foods you can consume almost as much as you'd like and eliminate the feelings of hunger, fatigue, and depression that often accompany other less satisfying calorie-restricted diets.

This low-calorie, high-volume eating plan includes foods with a lot of water and fibrous bulk since both may increase your sense of fullness.

However, no food is completely banned, and calorie-packed foods can be enjoyed as long as you stick within the your calorie for the day.

Low energy-dense foods include:

- Fruit
- Vegetables
- Low-fat dairy
- Whole grains
- Beans
- Lean meat

The Volumetrics Diet promises a one- to two-pound weight loss each week, which is an amount considered healthy by most nutrition and fitness professionals. Then you can maintain the weight loss for as long as you stick with the plan, which includes exercise. *The Volumetrics Diet* also promises that it won't drive you to give up and fall back on bad habits.

Dieters are encouraged to aim for 30 to 60

minutes of exercise a day and to keep a record of what they've eaten as well as any physical activity they've performed. That way, any areas that may need special attention can be addressed.

MyFitnessPal.com is awesome & free

I can't say enough good things about the *MyFitnessPal.com* app and website. It's a free program that you can use on the website, on your smartphone, or both. It monitors your nutritional consumption and exercise and also gives you the information you will need to effectively burn body fat.

It shows you how to set a reasonable body weight goal, with one pound per week being the default goal for weight loss. Losing one pound per week is just about the perfect weight-loss rate, mostly because you can be sure that you're losing body fat and not body muscle. A weight loss of one pound per week also allows you to gradually step into a healthier lifestyle, which means the changes you make are more likely to be permanent.

To use the app, you enter some basic information and your desired body weight, and then you simply let *MyFitnessPal.com* calculate the normal breakdown amounts of carbs, protein, sugars, sodium, fats, and total calories that you should consume daily. Then you enter your exercise type and amount, which the app uses to formulate a plan that will work for you.

As you eat, you will enter the foods and the amounts into the program, which helps you keep track of exactly what you have eaten. More than 1 million foods are listed in the *MyFitnessPal.com* database, and the user also has the option to add a food to the database. In addition, a product scanner allows you to collect information about packaged foods.

While at first it might seem difficult to remember to enter everything you eat, you will become accustomed to the system within a couple of days. It takes a bit of effort at first, but once it becomes a habit, you'll begin to realize just how easy the system is to use on a daily basis.

One of the best things about this app is that it can help you resist eating foods that you can't "afford" in your daily caloric intake. It offers a great way to hold you accountable, which is usually the first step to effective weight loss.

MyFitnessPal.com has a great support community of like-minded people who can help you stay encouraged and motivated, which is usually half the battle when it comes to consistent weight loss. At the end of the day, however, comes the best part, when you click on "complete this entry" and the MyFitnessPal.com app tells you "continue to eat this way and you'll weigh _____ pounds in_____ weeks."

Some users benefit from spending only one week on the program to get a basic idea of exactly how eating habits and exercise affect body weight. Use the program whenever you feel you need it, or use it all the time. *MyFitnessPal* app is free.

🏃🏃

*R*unkeeper.com

Social support can be important when it comes to reaching a goal. Health and fitness goals are no exception to this rule. This is why *RunKeeper.com*, a mobile app, adds so much value for the advancement of healthier lifestyles.

RunKeeper.com allows you to track your workouts and share your journey with friends and co-workers through social media sites such as

Facebook and Google Plus. More and more employers are offering wellness incentives to their employees, and *RunKeeper* is one way to show you're working out to ensure you receive those incentive rewards.

The feature that differentiates *RunKeeper.com* from other apps and gadgets is its training plan option. The app offers specific workout plans for different types of aerobic exercise, including walking, running, and biking. *RunKeeper.com* can help you track time, distance, and calories burned, allowing you to keep track of your progress from week to week.

You can also find plans to help you lose weight and begin running programs perhaps for the first time. These options are less intimidating for those looking for an overall healthy lifestyle that includes some aspect of cardio exercise.

Have you ever wanted to have a personal trainer at your fingertips? *RunKeeper.com* is headed in this direction. It is looking to expand beyond running and physical activity into a broader spectrum of encouraging an overall healthy lifestyle. Jason Jacobs, the CEO of *RunKeeper*, has said that "over time, the goal is to evolve into a sort of personalized coach for our users, helping them make smarter decisions about their health and fitness."

Workout Guru Mark Rippetoe's guide to strength and fitness

Many fitness professionals consider Mark Rippetoe to be the leading source for workout and exercise information, and in his book *Starting Strength,* he provides the reader with straightforward and effective methods to grow stronger. This instructional book offers important time-tested basic principles for exercisers of various levels of ability and experience, plus, specific instructions for important exercises that can be performed safely and successfully.

In addition, many fitness professionals consider *Starting Strength* to be one of the most useful fitness guides available.

The second edition of *Starting Strength: Basic Barbell Training* has sold more than 80,000 copies. While the barbell training detailed throughout the book is primarily aimed at young athletes, the training has also been successfully applied to all people, including seniors, male and female, fit or flabby, sick or healthy, and weak or strong.

Many people across the world have used the simple biological principle of stress/recovery/adaptation, on which this method is based, to improve their performance, appearance, and quality of life.

Now, after years of testing and adjustment

with thousands of athletes in seminars all over the country, the third edition expands and improves on the previous teaching methods and biomechanical analysis. *Starting Strength: Basic Barbell Training* provides detailed instruction on every aspect of the basic barbell exercises.

What follows is a versatile workout that can be performed in a gym or at home with little or no equipment. This strength/bodybuilding workout is performed three days a week:

- Monday – workout 1
- Wednesday – workout 2
- Friday – workout 1
- Monday – workout 2
- Wednesday – workout 1
- Friday – workout 2

Each exercise below is easy for home or gym.

Workout 1:

1. Squats with body weight or additional weight if appropriate, 2-3 sets of 8-10 repetitions per set.

2. Push-ups (from knees if necessary), press 2-3 sets, 8-10 repetitions per set.

3. Pull-ups (standing on a chair or help from a workout friend if necessary) for 2-3 sets, 5-15 reps.

4. Pull-downs, 2-3 sets of 8-10 repetitions per set.

5. Chair dips or dip bars with or without assistance, 2-3 sets of 8-10 repetitions per set.

Workout 2:

1. Step-forward lunges with or without weight, 2-3 sets of 8-10 repetitions per set.

2. Step-backward lunges with or without weight, 2-3 sets of 8-10 repetitions per set.

3. Standing military press (improvise weights at home or with weights in the gym), 2-3 sets of 8-10 reps per set.

4. Standing forward bends or lower back extensions, 2-3 sets of 8-10 reps per set.

5. Crunches, 2-3 sets of 20-25 reps per set.

Rest a day between each workout and don't do any two workouts on back-to-back days. The two workouts will be alternating. After about eight weeks, your body will adapt to the program, so it's time to change it out – a new routine and exercises.

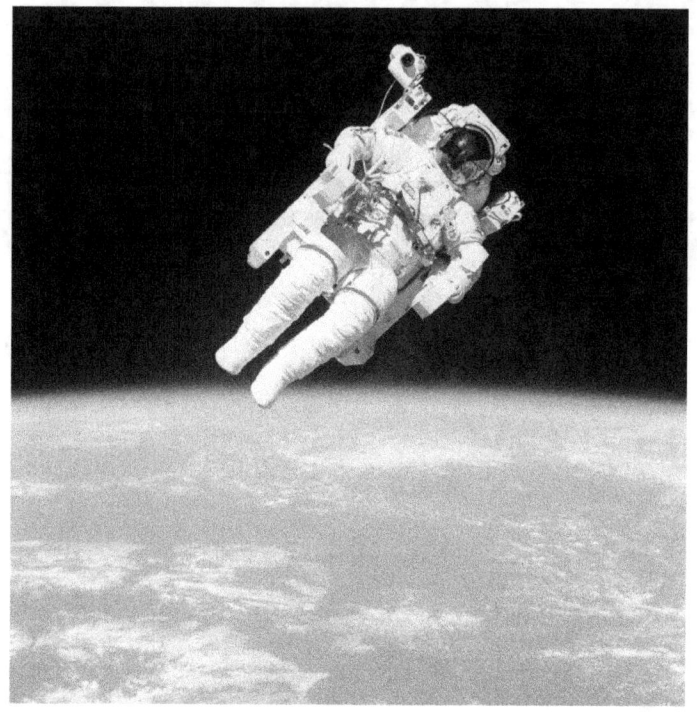

*S*itting kills, moving heals!

Author Joan Vernikos, PhD, a researcher at NASA, studied how weightlessness weakens astronauts' muscles and bones. In her book *Sitting Kills, Moving Heals,* she shows that a sedentary lifestyle contributes to poor health, obesity, and type II diabetes and that sitting still can kill you. She shows how health can be dramatically improved by low-intensity fitness movements that resist gravity.

Dr. Vernikos discovered that in weightlessness astronauts who are far fitter than the average adult seem to age rapidly because their muscles, bones, and overall health degenerate to levels usually seen in elderly people.

A lot of Americans sit or lie down much of the time, we drive to work, sit behind a desk, drive home, sit at the computer, watch TV, and read in bed. Dr. Vernikos found that standing up often, stretching, and walking are very healthy and were comparable to conventional exercise regimens for subjects who were otherwise inactive.

Along the road to your highest level of physical fitness, you are likely to have times of rapid progress, and, times of slower progress. Nevertheless, with your specific fitness goals in mind, and your commitment to consistency, your life-long fitness experience will be that of success.

END

www.ingramcontent.com/pod-product-compliance
Lightning Source LLC
Chambersburg PA
CBHW060508290526
45791CB00001B/315